Licensed to Thrive

A Mouth Owner's GPS to Vibrant Health & Innate Immunity

DR. FELIX LIAO, DDS

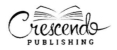

PUBLISHING

Licensed to Thrive
by Dr. Felix Liao

Cover Design by Khushnood - Klassic Designs
Copyright © 2020 by Dr. Felix Liao

ISBN: 978-1-948719-28-5 (P)
ISBN: 978-1-948719-29-2 (P-Color)
ISBN: 978-1-948719-30-8 (E)

Crescendo Publishing, LLC
300 Carlsbad Village Drive
Ste. 108A, #443
Carlsbad, California 92008-2999
1-877-575-8814

Dedication

Licensed to Thrive is dedicated to that new and growing breed of teeth-centered dentists turned Airway-centered Mouth Doctors® (AMDs) and Integrative Mouth Consultants—healthcare professionals who have dialed into the mouth's pivotal role in whole-body health.

Their cross-referrals and collaboration can help address the mouth as a root cause of pain and illness, and their combined expertise can help restore suffering patients back to a functional Whole.

Praise for License to Thrive

"In *Licensed to Thrive: A Mouth Owner's GPS to Vibrant Health,* Dr. Felix Liao reveals the interrelationships of everything from jaw structure, oral hygiene, the intestinal microbiome and cardiovascular health to environmental pollutants such as glyphosate (Round-Up). An interesting read from a biological dentist's perspective that helps connect the mouth not only with overall health but also the environment we live in."

James L. Wilson, ND, DC, PhD,
Adrenal Fatigue: The 21st Century Stress Syndrome

"In his delightful new book, *Licensed to Thrive*, Dr. Liao illustrates how we all have the capacity to achieve our full genetic potential, regardless of age. Optimizing our jaws and airway with the help of biomimetic oral appliance therapy, myofunctional therapy, physical therapy, and sound nutrition can help us achieve radiant health and longevity. Indeed, having a 'Holistic Mouth' supports our whole-body health and optimizes our sleep quality so that we can truly thrive."

Dr. Karen D. Cheng, MD,
Board-certified in Sleep Medicine & Neurology,
Laguna Hills, CA

"*Licensed to Thrive* book is about how become a smarter owner-operator of your mouth as a root cause of your illness and wellness. Your life quality and even your life depends on adopting Dr. Liao's advice."

Dr. Cristin Lewis, DDS
Nashville, TN

"I could not put it down. I read every word and hoped the knowledge would make a difference in me and my patients. Brilliantly written, easy to understand a MUST read for everyone."

Dr. Dawn Ewing, Executive Director,
IABDM.org

"Dr. Felix Liao's approach integrating mind-body-mouth can do more to upgrade health by addressing root causes instead of managing symptoms of chronic fatigue, pain, and degenerative diseases."

Dr. Sherry Salartash, DDS
Alexandria, VA

"Dr. Felix Liao has made bolstering your innate immunity entertaining, real, and educational. *Licensed to Thrive* is a must read for everyone who seeks wellness, longevity with life quality. Dr. Liao offers a sensible and do-able method to thrive in the face of fast and processed food, shrinking jaw structure, sleep apnea, and all the health disruptors from our 'civilized toxic world'. Make this the next book you read and the one that you give as gifts to all those whom you love."

Dr. Alvin Danenberg,
Periodontist,
Charleston, SC

"Bravo. you'd have heaven on earth if you read and implement this book! This time Dr. Liao provides a clear, concise road map connecting the dots between dental, airway, nutrition, and overall wellness in one book. I am excited to recommend this 'must have manual for proactive wellness' to EVERYONE, patients, and health care professionals alike. Dr. Liao's easy to understand style, relatable analogies makes implementing scientific evidence fun and relatable along the journey to life-long wellness."

Lauren Gueits, RDH, Bs,
Founder, Airway Health Solutions,
Northport, New York

"Breathing = Living. Breathing badly = Living badly. If you don't breathe, you don't live. Nutrition heals. Malnutrition kills. *Licensed to Thrive* book is about how become a smarter owner-operator of your mouth as a root cause of your illness and wellness. The quality AND quantity of your life depends on adopting Dr. Liao's sage advice. As a stage 4 cancer survivor who healed holistically, I know better than most what it takes to come back from devastation."

Dr. Teresa, M. Scott, DDS, MIABDM,
President, IABDM.org

"Dr. Liao is all about breathing, wellness and whole-health living which includes diet and nutrition. This book will help you discover your path to feeling better so you can live better. I recommend all of his books."

Dr. Leslie Haller, DMD,
Coral Gables, FL

"Dr. Felix Liao's new book is a timely call to action to put the 'care' back into health care. Dr. Liao does a wonderful job of showing that oral/airway health/nutrition is integral to whole body health. I encourage ALL health care professionals to address the mouth as a root causes of disease instead of treating symptoms. Dr. Liao's protocols and 'To-Do-Checklists' are easily implemented. *Licensed to Thrive* is now on my 'must-read' recommendation list!"

Dr. Ben Miraglia,
VP Clinical Affairs, Airway Health Solutions

"*License to Thrive* is definitely an important book for everyone who is interested in participating in their own health. This book takes dental care into 21st century...creating a new way dentistry will be understood and practiced. Dr. Liao's dedication, passion and vast clinical experience is exceptionally clear."

Dr. Nemie Sirilan, DDS,
Plainfield, NJ

"In his latest book, *Licensed to Thrive*, Dr. Liao teaches us how to reach our full genetic potential in mouth-oriented health and innate immunity. Mouth structure work creates the better version of ourselves naturally while we sleep. Dr. Liao seals the deal with nutrition that maximizes gut health. When it comes to gurus, I choose Dr. Felix Liao for his vast breadth of knowledge and experience in holistic/oral health."

Dr. Carolyn Schweitzer DDS,
Maynard, MA

"Dr. Liao exposes the greatest danger western civilization and Americans are facing: airway blockage and sleep apnea from deficient jaws and a steady diet of fast and processed foods. Dr. Liao's message is so simple and clear: you are the owner-operator of your mouth and CEO of your health. You need both a functional mouth Structure and a healthier mouth Style to have vibrant health. I have seen Felix's transformation over the past 25 years. Now I am starting mine with his guidance, because *Licensed to Thrive* is a universal GPS to a quality journey through life."

Dr. Michael D. Margolis, DDS,
Doctor of Integrative Medicine,
Mesa AZ

"Dr. Liao's *Thrive* has shed light on a host of cascading illnesses. Their root cause has been hidden in plain sight — Impaired Mouth Syndrome. Dr. Liao delivers breakthrough technology of our century in this book. Read it to turn from suffering to vibrant health. Get help as explained, and you will be well again naturally."

Mark DeEulio,
Alternative Healthcare Consultant

Contents

Licensed to Thrive:
A Mouth Owner's GPS To Vibrant Health & Innate Immunity

Introduction

"Disease enters through the mouth."

~ Chinese proverb

You are not only what you eat, but also HOW you eat, sleep, and live. Your mouth is the source of your energy and the gateway to your whole-body health. *Licensed to Thrive* is your "driver's training" on how to own and operate your mouth toward vibrant health naturally and away from obesity, diabetes, cancer, heart issues, or other killer diseases proactively.

Give your body what it needs, and it will thrive. What does your body need from you, its CEO? Refreshing sleep and nourishing eats are vital necessities, and both are mouth-mediated. *Licensed to Thrive* is a primer to build your overall health and innate immunity, starting with your mouth.

A primer is not a promise, but preparatory work to turn unpainted walls into finished rooms. This primer can transform you from an under-informed user-abuser of your mouth to a mindful owner-gardener. Is your body a greenhouse for sustainable wellness, or a tinderbox for inflammation and catastrophic illness?

Building health is an inside job, just like happiness, whereas fighting serious disease requires outside help. Do you prefer heroic fire-fighting to save your life or routine wellness-keeping to enjoy life? *Licensed to Thrive* shows the smarter way.

Do you feel like a sitting duck while killer diseases run wild all around you? The risk of COVID-19 infection severity and death compounds with underlying conditions—cardiovascular disease, diabetes, obesity, among others. What can you do besides wear a mask, wash your hands, and social distance?

The best defense to head off illness is a strong offense to turn on wellness. Sleep strengthens your innate immunity[1] that is "naturally present and is not due to prior sensitization to an antigen from, for example, an infection or vaccination." A structurally sound mouth supports airway and promotes deep sleep, while an impaired mouth collapses airway and disrupts sleep.

Your mouth is the main driver between serious illness or thriving wellness. This is my point: sound sleep and sensible eating can slow degeneration and empower your immune SWAT team.

Seventy percent of your immune system resides in the gut[2], while 100% of your gut health hinges on how you operate your mouth. *Licensed to Thrive* is your new GPS to vibrant health and innate immunity starting with a structurally sound mouth sensibly used.

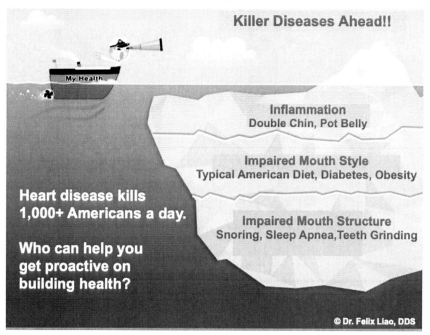

Your mouth can bolster or weaken your innate immunity and overall health in two major ways: Structure (physical equipment) and Style (usage).

- An impaired mouth Structure can contribute to recurring pain, fatigue, teeth grinding, and sleep apnea from choked airway. Oxygen deprivation is a major source of the degeneration of your heart, brain, and whole-body health—read *Six-Foot Tiger Three-Foot Cage*[3] and *Early Sirens*[4], or see Impaired Mouth Syndrome & Holistic Mouth Solutions next for a brief overview.
- An impaired mouth **Style** does not know when to stop eating, what's good for health, or how to eat for wellness. This is the root of obesity, inflammation, heart disease, diabetes, cancer, and degenerative killer diseases. Either deficiency or excess can mean health troubles.

Licensed to Thrive combines sound mouth "Structure" with sensible eating "Style" for Holistic Mouth Solutions to turbocharge your total health.

Just as you have your lifestyle, you also have a mouth style—how you use your mouth to eat, drink, and relate to people and Planet Earth. What you eat is only a part of Holistic Mouth Style, which is also how fast you eat, how often, in what mood, at what time, and how to enjoy eating without getting overfed and under-nourished. How much is enough, and how can you avoid overeating?

Eating a perfect diet only gets you so far, however, because oxygen is not optional and sleep apnea is rampant. You need *both* a functional mouth Structure *and* a healthier mouth Style to keep America's leading killer diseases away.

Leading Causes of Death, 2017

US Centers for Disease Control & Prevention

Dr. Liao: Mouth contributions include diet, infections, and airway obstruction.

1. Heart disease	23.0 %
2. Cancer	21.3 %
3. Accidents (unintentional injuries)	6.0 %
4. Chronic lower respiratory diseases	5.7 %
5. Stroke (cerebrovascular diseases)	5.2 %
6. Alzheimer's disease	4.3 %
7. Diabetes	3.0 %
8. Influenza and pneumonia	2.0 %
9. Kidney diseases	1.8 %
10. Intentional self-harm (suicide)	1.7 %

© Dr. Felix Liao, DDS

Impaired mouth Structure and untrained mouth Style combine to drive America's leading causes of death.

If your journey through life is a road trip, then a structurally impaired mouth is bad equipment turning your car into a "lemon." Worse yet, today's roads are increasingly paved with nutritional landmines from processed and fast foods that have been tampered with. Why wait until you have to sleep with a machine or rely on walkers, medications, catheters, and diapers? It's smarter to get "licensed" now.

From Symptom Management to Root-Cause Solutions

Do you have aches and pains that keep coming back, or creeping weight gain that won't budge no matter what you try? Why, and what will happen next if nothing changes? This is where you come in as the CEO-owner of your health.

Behind most entrenched symptoms lurks an impaired mouth Structure or Style, or both. Attending to one but not the other means falling short of feeling well. These are the patterns I've noticed over the years:

A. Symptom Management + Impaired mouth Structure => Limited Results

B. Symptom Management + Impaired mouth Style => Wasted Money

C. Impaired mouth Structure + Style => Escalating Health Troubles and Costs

D. Functional mouth Structure + sensible mouth Style => Thriving Wellness

Which pattern fits your experience? The first three describe nearly all my new patients. For example, Kim S. came to see me about her fatigue and neck and shoulder pain after reading *6-Foot Tiger 3 Foot-Cage*. Tall and lanky, she'd always eaten healthy. "I always felt better after doing nutrition, yoga, chiro, and Thai massage, but there's something beyond their reach. I just can't believe a mouthpiece could make such a dramatic difference," Kim commented 10 days after starting oral appliance for her impaired mouth Structure.

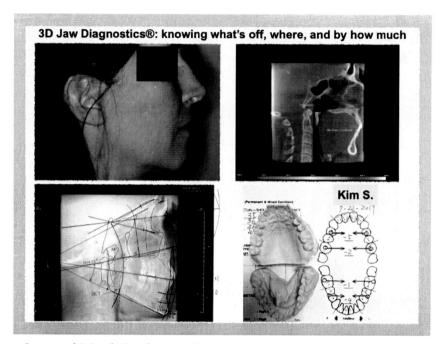

Impaired Mouth Syndrome of Kim S.: Airway in the red-black (dangerously narrow) zone because both jaws are underdeveloped. Healthy eating alone cannot fix this problem.

Kim's mouth Structure was the source of her recurring pain and fatigue—her case fits into pattern A. At 30% of low comfort, her airway would have been a serious health liability ahead. What if she had not eaten healthy?

Many patients with heart disease and sleep apnea are in pattern C, already burdened with pot bellies, double chins, oxygen debt, and energy deficit. This builds health risks and breeds runaway inflammation.

Personal Health Keeping: Mouth, Sleep, Immunity

Thriving health and illness recovery both require the same basics: oxygen, sleep, nutrition, shelter, mental peace, and social-emotional connections. The difference is *when* healthcare is delivered: reactive after a fire rages, or proactive before sparks catch fire. Are you for a ton of cure or an ounce of prevention?

A ventilator is at the end of a row of dominos. How can you keep the first piece standing strong, and what'd that be? Why get oxygen in a hospital when you can get it with an oral appliance and sleep in your own bed? You can fight for your life in the ICU or stay well with Holistic Mouth Solutions as first-line personal practice at home. Here's a brief look at the science.

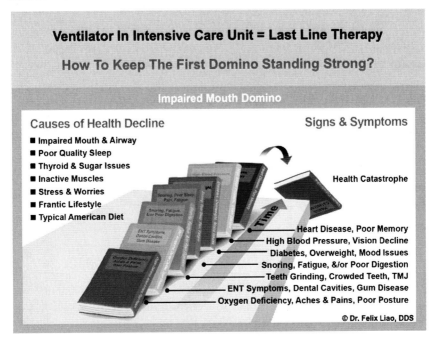

First, impaired mouth Structure leads to poorer sleep, and now, this 2019 study[5] from Germany connects sleep with immunity: "Indeed, sleep affects various immune parameters, is associated with a reduced infection risk, and can improve infection outcome and vaccination responses. Prolonged sleep deficiency (e.g., short sleep duration, sleep disturbance) can lead to chronic, systemic low-grade inflammation and is associated with various diseases that have an inflammatory component, like diabetes, atherosclerosis, and neuro-degeneration."

Simply put, poor sleep means poorer health and more infections.

Beware, teeth grinders[6] and people with tooth prints on the sides of the tongue[7].

Secondly, unhealthy mouth Style contributes to obesity and diabetes, which carry serious consequences. "Diabetes has rapidly emerged as a major comorbidity for COVID-19 severity," states this 2020 French study[8] on 1317 hospitalized patients, 88.5% with Type 2 diabetes. It concludes, "BMI [body mass index[9]] was positively and independently associated with tracheal intubation and/or death [outcome] within 7 days." It links said outcome to these prior conditions:

- Treated obstructive sleep apnea: Odds Ratio[10] (OR) 2.80
- Microvascular (diabetic) complications: OR 2.54
- Age: OR 2.48

You can't change your chronological age, but you can control obesity and diabetes to reduce COVID-19 severity by getting "licensed" to thrive.

Hello, Holistic Mouth Style

How much is too much at lunch, dinner, Thanksgiving, or an all-you-can-eat buffet? How much butter and syrup should you put on your pancake or waffle? Why are diet books perennial bestsellers?

The short answer: few of us are taught how to eat in this land of milk and honey and abundance.

The longer answer is your body has been coping with all the stressors and health disruptors baked into the American food chain and lifestyle—see chapters 1-4.

Holistic Mouth Style connects your mouth with your 3-part human brain—reptilian, emotional, and cognitive—to turn stress eating and toxin ingestion into pleasurable health building. Holistic Mouth Style thus includes both:

- Eating Well: avoiding hyper-processed foods that come with added sugars, fats, salt, synthetic chemicals, herbicides, preservatives, etc., and choosing organic, sustainably grown foods free of additives, antibiotics, and injected hormones.
- Eating Right: knowing how much to eat, how fast, in what combinations, at what temperature, and in what mood; knowing when stress-eating has got you; when to stop at "Just right" and still feel fully satisfied.

Holistic Mouth Style is a necessary wellness skill to keep your waist lean, gut clean, and inflammation down. Growing old is inevitable, but growing old in failing health is living hell.

Failing Health: A Sneak Peek

Graying of U.S. Bankruptcy[11] (2018) reports "an almost five-fold increase in the percentage of older persons in the US bankruptcy system." Low income and healthcare costs are the main culprits. I see illiteracy on how to eat as another.

"Growing old is a pathetic thing. It is full of limitation and reduction. It happens to us all, I know; but I think that it might not have to," says Enzo, an extraordinary dog with wisdom to share with us humans and the narrator in Garth Stein's novel *The Art of Racing in the Rain*[12]. Here, old and lying in a puddle of his own urine waiting for his owner, Enzo laments: *"I'm old. And while I'm very capable of getting older, that's not the way I want to go out.... Shot full of pain medication and steroids to reduce the swelling in my joints. Vision fogged with cataracts. Puffy, plasticky packages of Doggy Depends stocked in the pantry...my body deteriorating, disintegrating around me, dissolving until there's nothing left but...all sorts of cables and tubes feeding what remains."*

The prospect is nasty and the ending is ugly if impaired mouth Structure goes undiagnosed and Style unchecked. How do you want to go out? Take Enzo's experience to heart.

Unlike Enzo, however, YOU are the driver of your own destiny. YOU can turn away from pathetic aging—with the right "driver's training" to fully enjoy eating without crashing your health, experience bliss, and die in peace.

The Road Forks Here: Crash or Thrive

Healthcare isn't something you buy, such as "health insurance" to cover the cost of drugs and surgery. Healthcare is the care you put into your body, not a free lunch from your government or a card from your employer.

Health is a set of capabilities you cultivate in yourself with your lifestyle and nourish with your mouth style. Your doctor can be a guide, but not a "provider" to fill your energy tank.

Energy is the difference between illness-wellness and death-life. You can drain and deplete your life energy by overworking, over-partying, or over-indulging until you drop. Or, you can replete it with living right, sleeping well, and eating smarter to go the full distance in good order. *Licensed to Thrive* shows you how to renew that life energy in doable baby steps. "Thrive" here means:

- Having all the energy to support your life, resist infections, and heal faster.
- Reaching into deep sleep to restore your body from daily wear and tear.
- Rising above the old patterns of overeating, stress eating, and binging.
- Enjoying a better outcome from your diet and exercise.
- Getting better medical-dental checkups and healthier bio-markers.
- Finding the spring in your steps, gas in your tank, sunshine in your heart, and glow on your face.

"Thrive" is baked into your youth, but how can you keep thriving after age 39? That's where fixing your impaired mouth Structure and Style as your energy source comes in. *Licensed to Thrive* shows you what you want to do before your health abandons you.

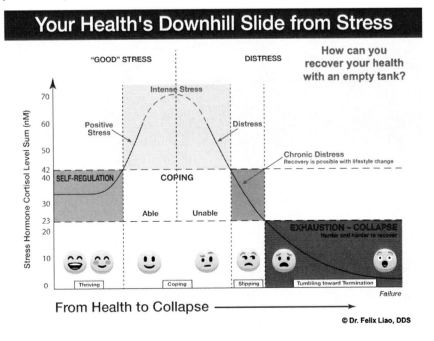

Finally, a catastrophic illness (a stroke, cancer, Alzheimer's) can derail your financial planning and drain your retirement income. The earlier you get "licensed to thrive," the safer your health in retirement.

"Give a man a fish, and you feed him for one meal" is a well-known Taoist wisdom. "Teach him how to fish, and you feed him for a lifetime."

Give people health insurance, and you help them get by. Get them licensed to thrive, and you empower their health for a lifetime.

Let's get started.

Author's Note About This Book

"Never believe that a few caring people can't change the world. For, indeed, that's all who ever have."

~ Margaret Mead

As a patient-consumer, you can and indeed will change your health and life by knowing Impaired Mouth Syndrome and Holistic Mouth Solutions. As a parent, you can similarly bring out your children's peak potential.

As an Airway-centered Mouth Doctor and Integrative Mouth Consultant, you can and indeed will change the health and life of your patients by diagnosing Impaired Mouth Syndrome and delivering Holistic Mouth Solutions.

This book began as a series of chairside chats with patients seeking root-cause solutions for their aches and pains, fatigue, teeth grinding, infections, and various puzzling health troubles over the past 25 years. It ends as a primer on what you can do to help your whole-body health thrive as a "licensed" owner-operator of your mouth.

Licensed to Thrive is not another diet book and nutrition plan, but instead an introspective look at Impaired Mouth Syndrome as a larger problem, and Holistic Mouth Solutions as a root-cause answer. The concepts and connections are so new that this book is written for patients-consumers, integrative healthcare professionals, and dentists alike.

In the interest of brevity, the evidence I present in this book is meant to be representative, not exhaustive. My point is not to "snow" you with lots of studies, but to show breakthrough outcomes with sound mouth structure and sensible eating style.

If you are a consumer who just wants to know the headline and the bottom lines, simply read in this order: the Introduction, the starting paragraphs, the slides, and the bullet points at the end of each chapter, then chapters 21-25, and the Afterword. For reading efficiency, I recommend that you read through each chapter before checking the hyperlinked references.

Video testimonials by patients whose cases appear in this book are available online—see Resources.

Licensed to Thrive is also written to support the emerging new breed of Airway-centered Mouth Doctor® (AMD) and Integrative Mouth Consultants who are working together to treat Impaired Mouth Syndrome to make their patients well. This book works as an educational supplement for patients on how to eat before and during epigenetic oral appliance therapy.

This book's main focus is on you as the owner-operator of your mouth. You can see your dentist to fix toothaches or prevent them. Now, you can see an AMD or Holistic Mouth Consultant to give your body what it needs to thrive: wide-open airway, deep restorative sleep, and smarter eating. In short, your body works when your mouth is:

1. Cleaned up (free of silent infections and toxins), consistent with biological dentistry;
2. Well-developed structurally to remove airway obstruction as a source of chronic pain, fatigue, and premature aging;
3. Used wisely and proactively by its owner-operator to minimize gut inflammation, obesity, diabetes, cardiovascular diseases, cancer, Alzheimer's, and other killer diseases.

Nothing herein should be taken or mistaken for diagnosing or treating any specific disease or infection. See your healthcare professionals for individualized advice. Some people may have difficulty adopting Holistic Mouth Style successfully because of undiagnosed addiction disorders with smoking, alcohol, and sugar.

They should see a qualified medical professional or counselor for treatment.

Medications, body work, supplements, meditations, surgery, etc. all have a place in healthcare, but first thing first: deep sleep with a wide-open airway. The main thread of this book has these two interwoven strands: impaired mouth Style (not knowing how to eat for health) and Structure (choked airway from deficient jaws).

I will be posing many questions to connect your mind with my reasoning. Try to answer them as if we were having a chairside chat. You'll learn more this way. Knowing *why* can be an impetus to change health behavior. Knowing sugar's addictive and destructive power has helped me unhook from my sweet tooth.

You can eat your way into agonizing illness or thriving wellness. The mouth is where you can ruin or build your health. Here's to your shift from survive to thrive!

Dr. Felix K. Liao, DDS, MAGD, ABGD, MIABDM
Diplomate, American Sleep and Breathing Academy
Falls Church, Virginia

Impaired Mouth Syndrome and Holistic Mouth Solutions

"Everybody has a plan until they get punched in the mouth."

~ Mike Tyson,
Heavyweight Boxing Champion[1]

Health is a set of bodily functions based on structure. Poor form means weaker functions and thus poorer health.

An impaired mouth Structure comes with crowded teeth jammed into short and narrow jaws with jaw joint dysfunctions. Worse yet, smaller jaws force the tongue into the throat to block the airway. An impaired mouth Structure can still eat, drink, and talk, but it comes with a whole bunch of medical, dental and mood symptoms which I named Impaired Mouth Syndrome[2].

Impaired Mouth Syndrome's far-reaching consequences are sorely missing on the radars of nearly all doctors, dentists, and patients as of 2020. The following is a list of the more frequent symptoms of Impaired Mouth Syndrome.

Impaired Mouth Syndrome Score

Mouth	Score	Body	Score
Snoring, morning dry mouth	0 1	Gasping or choking in sleep	0 1
Teeth grinding, jaw	0 1	Neck, shoulder, or back pain; headaches	0 1
Mouth breathing, chapped lips	0 1	Erectile dysfunction or PMS	0 1
Persistent/wandering dental sensitivity	0 1	High blood pressure, heart disease	0 1
Gum recession and/or redness	0 1	Diabetes type 2, bloating after meals	0 1
Clicking/locking jaw joints, zigzag jaw opening	0 1	Weight gain, pot belly; acid reflux	0 1
Morning headache and/or sore jaws	0 1	Daytime sleepiness, fatigue	0 1
Deep overbite or underbite (weak chin)	0 1	Senile memory, ADD/ADHD	0 1
Frequent cavities or broken/chipped teeth	0 1	Frequent colds, flu, and skin disorders	0 1
Teeth prints on the sides of the tongue	0 1	Obstructive sleep apnea from a sleep test	0 1
Bony outgrowth on palate or inside lower jaw	0 1	Stuffy/runny nose, scratchy/itchy throat	0 1
Sunken lips and reverse smile curve (sad)	0 1	Forward head: ears ahead of shoulders	0 1
History of teeth extractions for braces	0 1	Waking up to urinate more than once	0 1
Bulge under lower jaw, double chin	0 1	Large neck size (M>17, W>15)	0 1
History of lots of dental work + medical symptoms	0 1	Poor digestion and elimination	0 1
Malocclusion (crowded teeth)	0 1	Depression, anxiety, grouchiness	0 1
Total Score		Total Score	

www.HolisticMouthSolutions.com

The higher your score, the more likely your structurally-impaired mouth is undermining your whole-body health. One single "Yes" is enough to suffer from Impaired Mouth Syndrome, as in a medical diagnosis of obstructive sleep apnea.

Holistic Mouth Solutions Fix Impaired Mouth Syndrome

I define a Holistic Mouth as one that is structurally fit to support whole-body health through Alignment, Breathing, Circulation, Digestion, Energy, and Sleep.

A Holistic Mouth has fully developed jaws, with room for all 32 natural teeth to line up straight naturally in the absence of health disruptors. A wide-open airway to support sleep and supply all the oxygen as needed comes with a holistic mouth.

Imagine a sharp thorn in your shoe, and you cannot take off the shoe. You'd have to compensate by walking abnormally, and soon pain shows up in your low back or neck. An impaired mouth structure is a huge thorn to your body because the mouth mediates the body's top survival reflexes: breathing and eating.

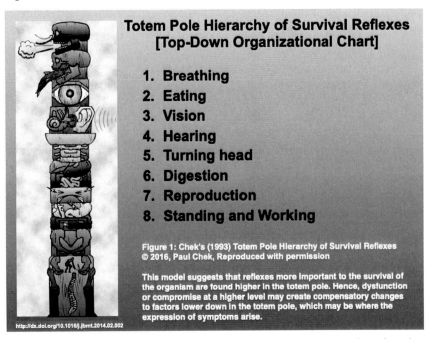

Totem Pole Hierarchy of Survival Reflexes [Top-Down Organizational Chart]

1. **Breathing**
2. **Eating**
3. **Vision**
4. **Hearing**
5. **Turning head**
6. **Digestion**
7. **Reproduction**
8. **Standing and Working**

Figure 1: Chek's (1993) Totem Pole Hierarchy of Survival Reflexes © 2016, Paul Chek, Reproduced with permission

This model suggests that reflexes more important to the survival of the organism are found higher in the totem pole. Hence, dysfunction or compromise at a higher level may create compensatory changes to factors lower down in the totem pole, which may be where the expression of symptoms arise.

http://dx.doi.org/10.1016/j.jbmt.2014.02.002

Top-down organizational chart of the human body, reproduced with permission.

Two Common Clues

Many of the symptoms listed above defy conventional treatment, which leads to higher cost, lower quality of life, and more frustration. Examples include pain returning after chiropractic adjustments or massages, or teeth grinding despite night guard, or teeth bunching up again after braces come off. That's what happens when the treatment misses the root cause—a structurally impaired mouth in this case.

Crowded lower front teeth and Liao's Sign are two common clues of an impaired mouth Structure.

Dental crowding stems from deficient jaw development—not enough bone volume, akin to not enough seats on the bus for all 32 "kids" (teeth) to get on. Having adult teeth extracted for braces and spaces closed further aggravates a structurally impaired mouth. This subtractive approach results in neck pain and airway obstruction that defy standard treatment.

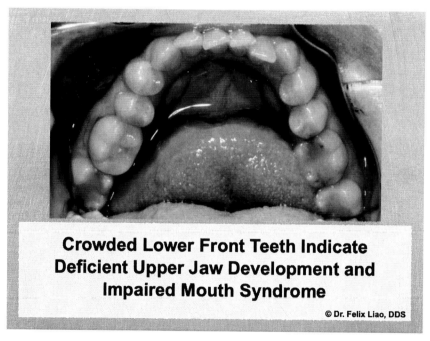

Crowded Lower Front Teeth Indicate Deficient Upper Jaw Development and Impaired Mouth Syndrome

© Dr. Felix Liao, DDS

Good development means the maxilla (upper jaw) should be wider so the lower teeth can fit into the uppers like a foot into a shoe without strain and pain. Crowded lower front teeth reflect an undersized "toe box" in the maxilla's front end.

Deficient jaw development also results in flat mid-face (Liao's Sign) and/or a weak chin. Liao's Sign is an experience-based observation that a narrow airway comes with a maxilla that failed to thrive (grow) forward. Underdeveloped maxilla is a much-overlooked source of many aches and pains resistant to medications, massage, and neck adjustments. Pain and fatigue often go down or go away completely with redevelopment.

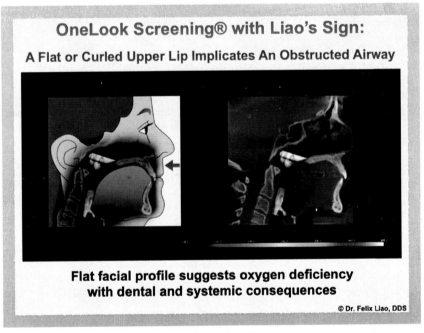

OneLook Screening® with Liao's Sign:

A Flat or Curled Upper Lip Implicates An Obstructed Airway

Flat facial profile suggests oxygen deficiency with dental and systemic consequences

© Dr. Felix Liao, DDS

Red arrow points to flat upper lip in the slide above and curled upper lip below.

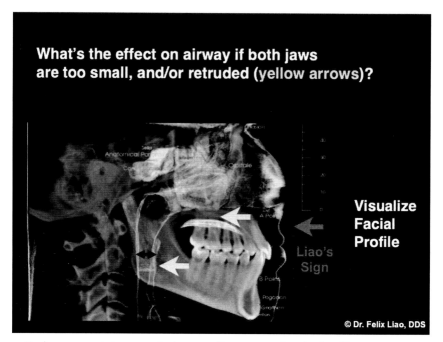

Red arrow points to curled upper lip, suggesting lack of bony support from retruded upper jaw (yellow arrow, opposite of protruded), which then retrudes the lower jaw and the tongue (yellow arrow) to narrow the airway (black arrows).

Airway is connected to jaws because of the functional space between the two jaws reserved for the tongue. Deficient jaws mean deficient oral space for the tongue, and the tongue is then driven into the throat, blocking oxygen delivery.

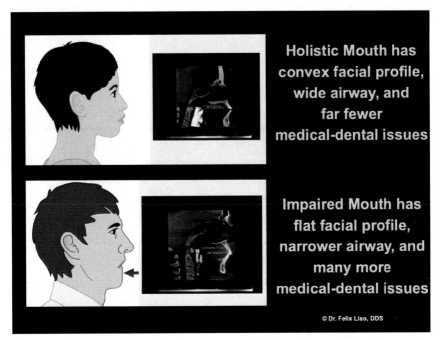

Holistic Mouth has convex facial profile, wide airway, and far fewer medical-dental issues

Impaired Mouth has flat facial profile, narrower airway, and many more medical-dental issues

© Dr. Felix Liao, DDS

A Holistic Mouth has sufficient jaw development and wide-open airway (white in the color scale). An Impaired mouth has deficient jaws, flat cheekbones and/or weak chin (red arrow), and likely crowded teeth and narrower airway (green-yellow-red).

Subtraction Orthodontics: A Double Whammy

How can you straighten bunched- up teeth in under-sized jaws efficiently? In the "dark ages" before WholeHealth linking teeth-jaws-alignment-airway, one answer was to extract some adult teeth and closing the spaces with braces. I call this treatment subtraction orthodontics because it makes the jaws already too small with crowded teeth even smaller.

The problem: the tongue was not made correspondingly smaller.

The result is a miserable patient with straight teeth and a double whammy: a more severe form of Impaired Mouth Syndrome often with wide-spread pain and fatigue, and twice the treatment to reopen the spaces lost to extractions at 3 to 5 times the cost.

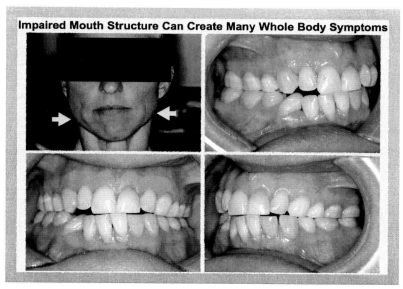

One case of subtraction orthodontics with 4 adult premolars extracted (1 in each quadrant). This results in teeth grinding, aches and pains, and Impaired Mouth Syndrome. Note canted mandible (yellow arrows) and slanted lip line.

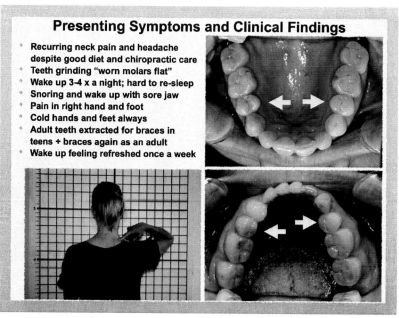

Subtraction orthodontic case and presenting symptoms; yellow arrows point to single premolar in each quadrant instead of 2.

Subtraction orthodontics goes against full jaw development to genetic potential.

Holistic Mouth with Full Jaw Development

A structurally impaired mouth means dental-facial development has fallen short of full genetic potential. Subtraction orthodontics aggravates deficient jaw development further. The great news: epigenetic oral appliance now makes jaw redevelopment possible at any age, provided enough sound natural teeth are present and a bone-building diet is followed.

A Holistic Mouth with fully developed jaws is a root-cause solution to many symptoms of Impaired Mouth Syndrome—see Forward for Healthcare Professionals next. Holistic Mouth Solutions can bring out your best look, peak performance, and life quality by making your mouth structurally sound to support whole-body health as follows:

A. Oral appliances designed with 3D Jaw Diagnostics®: an established method to identify what's off, where, and by how much in the two jaws to custom-design oral appliances for targeted correction (of the 3-foot cage) to promote sleep and remove oral contributions to chronic aches and pains and fatigue.

B. Mouth-body alignment: body work, chiropractics, cranio-sacral therapy, postural-restoration physical therapy, acupuncture, myofunctional therapy (physical therapy of the tongue, lips, and throat muscles), as needed.

C. Holistic Mouth Style: the new proactive wellness skill of how to eat to build health, promote sleep, reduce inflammation, and bolster immunity, as shown in this book.

The earlier the diagnosis and treatment, the easier the process and the better the outcome. The next slides show how 3D Jaw Diagnostics® and Holistic Mouth Solutions helped a 9-year-old with Impaired Mouth Syndrome.

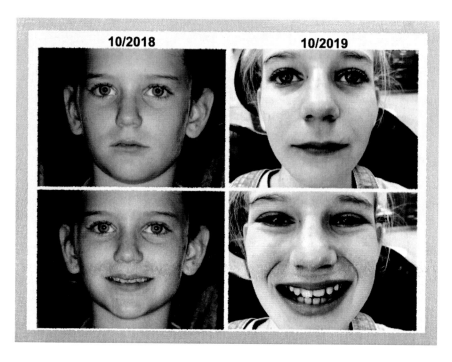

10/2018   10/2019

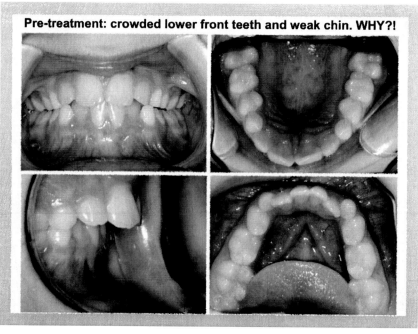

Pre-treatment: crowded lower front teeth and weak chin. WHY?!

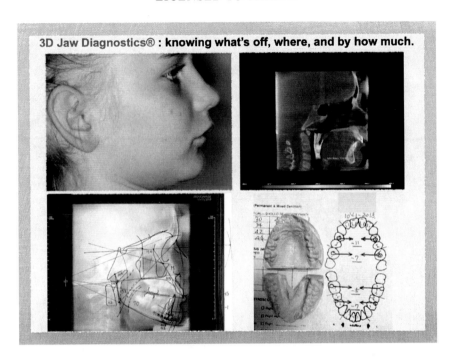

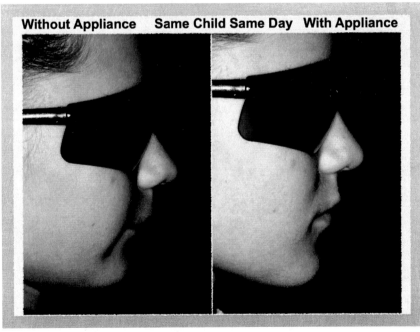

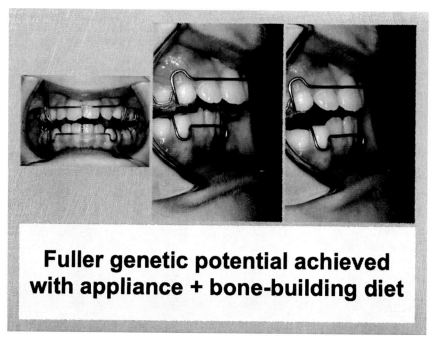

**Fuller genetic potential achieved
with appliance + bone-building diet**

*Above and below: Dr. Liao's Start Thriving Appliance™,
US and international patents pending.*

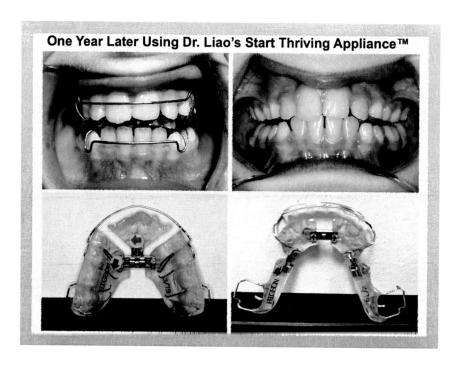

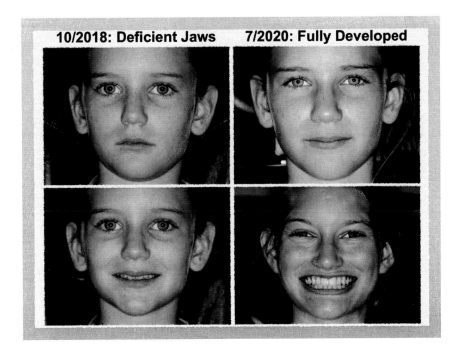

10/2018: Deficient Jaws   **7/2020: Fully Developed**

This young patient has wind in her developmental sail because her mom follows the Nourishing Traditions Diet of Weston A. Price Foundation. There's no congestion in her upper airway from typical American "junk food"—see chapter 18 and 23.

As a parent, you can bring out the full genetic potential of your child's dental-facial development with early recognition, 3D Jaw Diagnostics®, and timely Holistic Mouth Solutions.

As an adult long past your growth years, you can still reclaim your health by taking out the thorn of Impaired Mouth Syndrome using *Start Thriving Appliance™* paired to a bone-building diet, as shown in *Licensed to Thrive*.

Foreword for Healthcare Professionals on WholeHealth Integration

"Oral health is more than healthy teeth."

~ David Satcher, MD, US Surgeon General,
Oral Health America 2000[1]

The mouth is a critical infrastructure for airway and sleep, and thus a basic necessity for health maintenance and recovery. A fully functional mouth goes far beyond chewing and smiling to support whole-body health. Yet the idea of a functional Holistic Mouth is gravely missing in 2020 healthcare.

Simply put, a Holistic Mouth supports whole-body health, while an impaired mouth creates a collection of symptoms known as Impaired Mouth Syndrome that defy standard treatment: snoring, sleep apnea, chronic pain, fatigue, airway obstruction, jaw joint clicks/pops, teeth grinding, depression, anxiety, brain fog, sympathetic dominance, infection susceptibility, and more.

The rising tide of Impaired Mouth Syndrome, obesity, and sleep apnea points to the sore need for functional mouth doctors. It's time to break out of the silo mentality built into our respective training. Privately, medical doctors tell me, "I know I'm supposed to look inside the patient's mouth, but I have no idea what to look for." Historically, dental schools train dentists to be good tooth doctors. That's why the mouth is missing in the medical-dental divide.

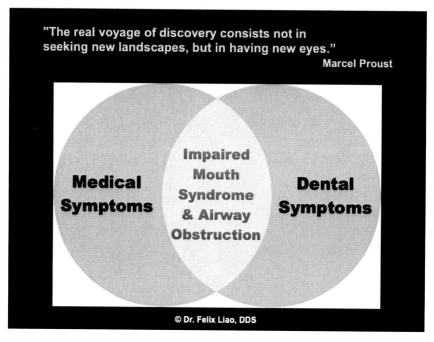

"The real voyage of discovery consists not in seeking new landscapes, but in having new eyes."
Marcel Proust

Medical Symptoms

Impaired Mouth Syndrome & Airway Obstruction

Dental Symptoms

© Dr. Felix Liao, DDS

Ninety-three percent of dentists and healthcare professionals (HCPs) in my seminars suffer from Impaired Mouth Syndrome just like their patients, but the answer is not widely known yet. Here's an email from a surgeon's wife:

> "I noticed you specialize in mouth and nose and better breathing. My husband is a CT [cardiac-thoracic] surgeon. He has sleep apnea and snores very loud! About 20 years ago I made him get a sleep study. He had worn a CPAP all these years but as you know its pain to deal with. It's not comfortable sometimes he takes it off snores loud and also he has to clean [it] every day. We saw an ad on tv for Inspire and went to Jefferson for a consult. The surgeon said his sleep apnea was too mild for that and said my husband needed a septo-

plasty and turbinate. He had that surgery it was one week of hell he still recovering and he still has to wear the CPAP and he still snoring so really it didn't resolve anything!! Anyway, I just want to find out what your solutions are!?"

My heart goes out to the surgeon and his wife. He likely suffers from undiagnosed Impaired Mouth Syndrome. His case reveals the limitations of staying "in the box," and the need for another approach—WholeHealth Integration.

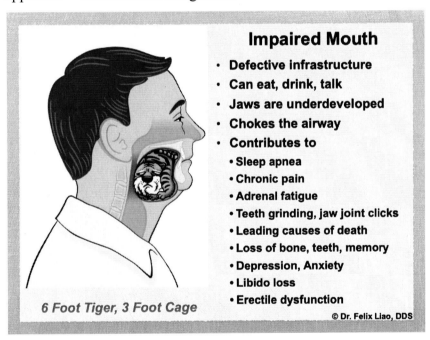

Impaired Mouth

- **Defective infrastructure**
- **Can eat, drink, talk**
- **Jaws are underdeveloped**
- **Chokes the airway**
- **Contributes to**
  - **Sleep apnea**
  - **Chronic pain**
  - **Adrenal fatigue**
  - **Teeth grinding, jaw joint clicks**
  - **Leading causes of death**
  - **Loss of bone, teeth, memory**
  - **Depression, Anxiety**
  - **Libido loss**
  - **Erectile dysfunction**

6 Foot Tiger, 3 Foot Cage

© Dr. Felix Liao, DDS

WholeHealth Integration Brings Breakthrough Outcomes

WholeHealth simply recognizes that all parts of the body are seamlessly interconnected and coordinated. When one part falls short, the rest compensate and symptoms appear. Effective healthcare calls for more than symptom management.

WholeHealth Integration aims to restore each chronically ill patient back to a functional Whole with natural solutions—or least side effects, where possible. It answers this question: What else does this patient need besides my expertise to regain self-regulation?

Every chronically-ill patient needs a fully functional or holistic mouth—one that can support whole-body health with airway, sleep, and nutrition. The alternative is to put up with CPAP and live with Impaired Mouth Syndrome in frustration. The problems experienced by the surgeon and his wife can readily be solved with WholeHealth Integration—a platform for medical-dental collaboration among all HCPs.

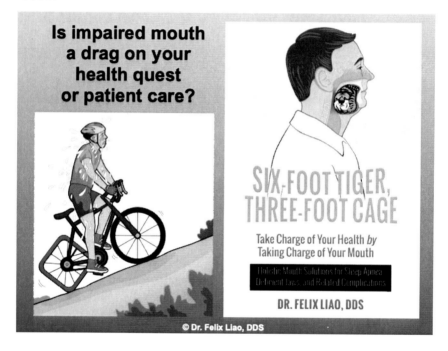

Care for health starts with alignment, breathing, circulation, digestion, and sleep to make energy (ABCDES). Inside the human body, there are no departmental lines.

Impaired mouth Structure is a much-overlooked health blocker. WholeHealth Integration can bring breakthrough outcomes by inter-disciplinary collaboration to deliver ABCDES to patients. The body responds readily when impaired mouth Structure is recognized and treated appropriately. Here's an actual case of another HCP who did just that.

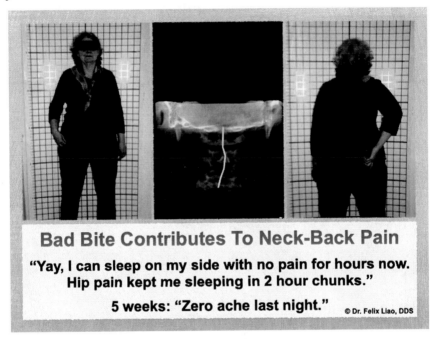

Bad Bite Contributes To Neck-Back Pain

"Yay, I can sleep on my side with no pain for hours now. Hip pain kept me sleeping in 2 hour chunks."

5 weeks: "Zero ache last night." © Dr. Felix Liao, DDS

"Can your oral appliance help me?" asked Miss Miller, age 67. Her hip was scheduled for joint replacement surgery that was shelved by COVID lockdown. Miss Miller was referred by a fellow HCP whose neck and back pain had resolved with oral appliances. Her presenting complaints and airway are shown in the slide below. Her airway was in the red-black (seriously narrow) zone that's 25% of the white (ideal) zone.

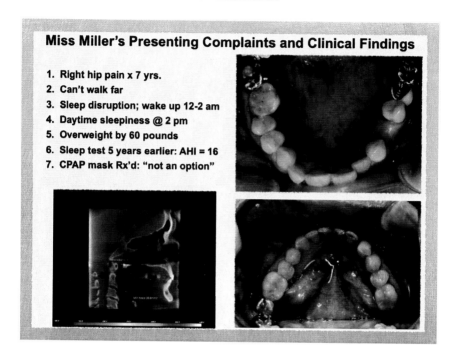

Miss Miller's Presenting Complaints and Clinical Findings

1. Right hip pain x 7 yrs.
2. Can't walk far
3. Sleep disruption; wake up 12-2 am
4. Daytime sleepiness @ 2 pm
5. Overweight by 60 pounds
6. Sleep test 5 years earlier: AHI = 16
7. CPAP mask Rx'd: "not an option"

Three weeks after starting oral appliance, Miss Miller emailed me: "My daytime exhaustion is abating with the oral appliance and the improved quality of sleep from it. This is very exciting because it has been happening for 4 years. I can say my hip pain is only intermittent now and I can trace it to times when I have overdone with the yoga or exercise. Now I am hopeful I can start to lose weight and add some more health improvement. Thank you!"

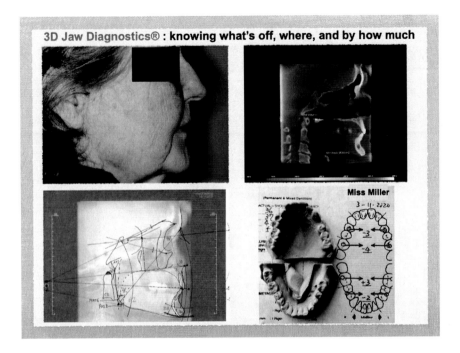

Not all oral appliances are created equal. This is a single upper appliance designed with the 3D Jaw Diagnostics® method. Miss Miller's hip pain had an oral contribution from her life-long cross bite from maxilla underdevelopment. See more of her progress in Afterword-2 for healthcare professionals.

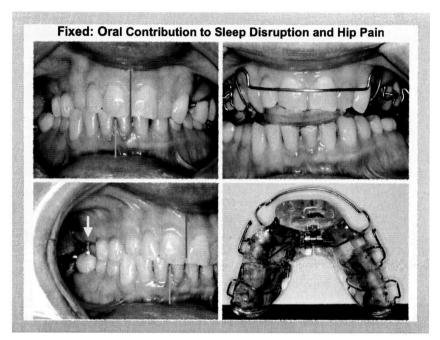

Fixed: Oral Contribution to Sleep Disruption and Hip Pain

Upper left: Discrepancy of dental mid-lines (blue for upper; orange for lower)

Lower left: Yellow arrow points to 3 crowns perpetuating cross bite from narrow maxilla

Upper and lower right: Dr. Liao's Start Thriving Appliance™, (US and international patents pending) designed with 3D Jaw Diagnostics® removes oral contributions to Miss Miller's hip pain.

Dental work (3 crowns in her right molars) perpetuated her cross bite and locked her into her hip pain. I did not know that at first, even as a when I was a tooth-centered dentist for a long time. But now, as a holistic mouth doctor, I know that misaligned upper and lower mid-lines is a frequent source of neck-shoulder-back pain.

"My hip pain is down from 10 to 1, and only once in a while when I overdo yoga," Miss Miller reports two months later. "I can get up from sitting without ouch. It used to hurt 20 minutes into a car ride, but I had a 6-hour road trip without any aching. My pain went down a notch when I stopped cheese, and yet another level when I stopped chips. Now I can sleep the whole night when I used to sleep in 2-hour chunks." See Resources for the link to her video testimonial.

This appliance offered Miss Miller a test drive and freed her body from her undiagnosed Impaired Mouth Syndrome (cross bite). The expander feature built into her appliance in combination with a bone-building diet can redevelop her deficient maxilla epigenetically in combination with a bone-building diet. Age does not matter, but the presence of sound teeth does.

Is undiagnosed Impaired Mouth Syndrome limiting your clinical success? WholeHealth Integration can help bring breakthrough results by removing Impaired Mouth Syndrome as a blocker to your patients' ability to self-regulate.

Chapter 1

Your Mouth, Your Health, Your Life

"If you have sleep apnea, heart disease, diabetes, obesity and many largely preventable diseases, you are much more likely to succumb to any type of infection, COVID-19 included. This is not rocket science but common sense."

~ Cecilia Wu, M.D.,
Anatomic, Forensic, and Cardiovascular Pathologist

Your mouth is a major driver of your illness or wellness. Your health depends on how you own and operate your mouth more than you can imagine. If you want good health, you'll need to take charge of your mouth. Let's see why first.

Every newborn grows from repeated cycles of sleeping and feeding. The rest of your body develops from the top downward. Your mouth is not just an opening with teeth for smiles. Your mouth is a vital organ foundational to your whole body and life quality.

How do health troubles start in the first place? Your mouth is the admission office between the outside and your inside. Imagine you are standing in chin-deep water in a pool or at the beach. One small wave can get you in big health trouble. The water level represents your internal inflammation and health risk for diabetes, obesity, heart disease, cancer, and other killer diseases. Your mouth is both the source and the solution.

You are not just what you eat; you are also how well you sleep and breathe. Your energy, immunity, healthcare costs, longevity, and life quality all depend greatly on your:

- Mouth Structure: Whether your jaws are well-formed to support airway and sleep;
- Mouth Style: How you eat for pleasure with wellness, or obesity with inflammation.

Thriving health requires both sound mouth Structure and Style. Your body prioritizes oxygen above food, medications, or supplements. This crucial point is gravely missing in healthcare still. Many patients and doctors have come to see me with straight, white, cavity-free teeth, clean gums, and a healthy lifestyle and eating habits, and still they fall short of feeling well. A good dental checkup is an important start, but it's only one part of a fully functional mouth that supports whole-body health with alignment, breathing, circulation, digestion, energy, and sleep.

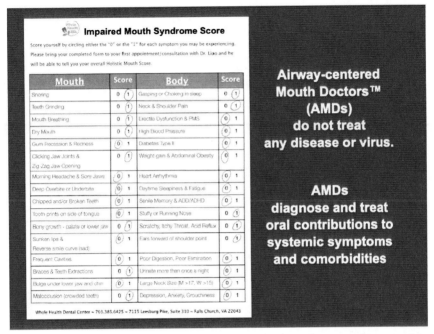

Impaired Mouth Syndrome Score of a super-high performing chiropractic doctor who works out, eats clean, stays lean, passes medical and dental check-ups, and still snores, grinds teeth, wakes up tired, and suffers neck-shoulder pain despite adjustments His pain level is zero after starting Start Thriving Appliance™ after 3-4 weeks..

Below the surface, your mouth is a vital infrastructure involved in whole-body health far beyond chewing and smiling. Health is a series of recurring functions, and we know functions follow form. What if the mouth is a defective infrastructure? Let's zoom out to look at the big picture first.

The mouth is big in whole-body health. Type "homunculus" into your search engine to see a body map based on the number of neurons devoted to each part. The mouth and the hands are disproportionately large—evidence that hand-to-mouth dominance is both a survival necessity and a path to illness or wellness.

Do you eat to live, or live to eat? Indulging your sweet tooth at will and not knowing how to eat for health can lead to nasty diseases like diabetes and cancer, as well as catastrophic events like a stroke or heart attack.

The mouth is your control switch to turn on illness or wellness. Once you've swallowed that mouthful, your gut can only react. Its reactions are either digestion and absorption, or indigestion and congestion leading to obesity and inflammation—the source of most killer diseases.

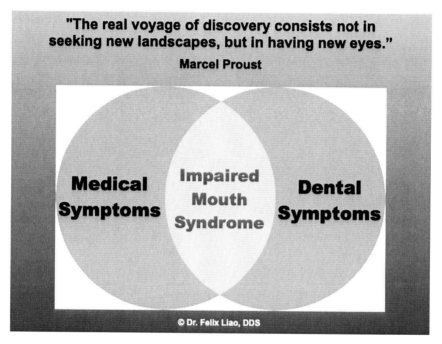

Impaired Mouth Syndrome in this book includes the medical, dental, and mental-emotional consequences of both impaired mouth Structure and Style. Impaired Mouth Syndrome in this book includes the medical, dental, and mental-emotional consequences of both impaired mouth structure and style, but it's not yet on the radars of most doctors, dentists, and healthcare professionals.

'My Cancer Has Come Back'

I can never forget this call from a new patient around 2005: "Dr. Liao? Hi, this is Helen. I really need to see you ASAP, because my cancer has come back. I had double mastectomy years ago, and the only thing I have not done is biological dentistry to make sure my teeth are not harming my health."

It took me a moment to regain my composure enough to reply, "I see you have done your homework, and my heart goes out to you. First, may I ask where your latest cancer is located?" Just above her collarbone, Helen said. She made an appointment but never came in. I've wondered about Helen ever since.

What might have helped Helen from recurrent cancer? I wonder what would have happened if she had cleaned up and straightened her mouth first. After all, the mouth is the start of the digestive system, and the lymphatics drain from the mouth down the neck toward the chest, not to mention airway and sleep.

Diet is typically the first change when a patient gets a cancer diagnosis. Why wait until the horse has left the barn? *Licensed to Thrive* is all about getting you to change your way of eating proactively—long before your immunity quits.

Colorectal cancer is the second most common type of cancer in women, and the third in men, and the fourth in mortality worldwide. "The liver is the most common site of metastasis in patients with colorectal cancer due to its anatomical situation regarding its portal circulation," reports this 2017 study[1]. "Median survival without treatment is < 8 months…and a survival rate at 5 years of 11% is the best prognosis."

Cancer, or any illness, is an outcome. Prognosis is poor if your liver gets "direct deposits" from colon cancer. When should you take control of the source? What are the causes? Among the many, there's no denying that oral contributions are big. For example, this 2012 study[2] found cancer death rate goes up 4.8 times with severe sleep apnea and 2 times with moderate sleep apnea.

You need your liver to live and to fight infections and cancer. What does it take to support your liver? It starts with the same requirement to eat and live healthy: deep sleep, wide-open airway, oxygen as needed, and a caring owner who avoids added sugar, alcohol overuse, junk food, and toxins.

Obesity, Gut Inflammation, and Killer Diseases

A patient who is a flight attendant came back 3 months later with 30 pounds lost. How did she do it? "I was furloughed during the COVID-19 lockdown, so I slept in more and ate 2 meals a day instead of 3."

She was also eating a bone-building diet (chapters 23-24) as part of her *Start Thriving Appliance™*, therapy, and she was sleeping deeper. This combination can be effective to reduce the risk of killer diseases.

"Obese patients have increased intensive care unit length of stay and are more likely to die in the hospital," reports a 2012 review[3] of research on the impact of obesity on the immune response to infection. "Further...obesity increases infection susceptibility in clinical settings."

Obesity means not only larger size, but also higher risk of infections and death. Obesity, Type 2 Diabetes, serious heart conditions, COPD, and chronic kidney disease increase the risk of severe illness from COVID-19 at any age, says U.S. CDC[4].

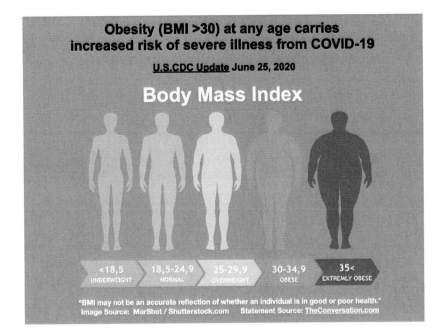

Historically, having enough to eat was the big challenge to survival. Today, obesity is "common, serious, and costly," says U.S.CDC[5]. More than 71% of Americans are overweight in 2020, over 40% are obese, and 18% severely obese. By 2030, obesity will strike one of every two Americans, and one of four will be severely obese, according to a 2019 study[6].

"I lived in Amsterdam for two years," one patient told me during her checkup. "You can always pick the Americans out of a crowd over there—they are the fat ones." We can see American eating style clearly through the lens of this Tunisian eighth grader attending summer school in Providence, RI. "I never saw so many tall buildings and fat people" was his answer when I asked for his first impressions of America.

How do so many get so fat? The short answer is clueless eating with an impaired mouth Style. Let's connect the mouth to obesity, sleep apnea, and killer diseases. First, impaired mouth **Style** contributes to inflammation as follows:

- **Obesity fans inflammation.** "As a risk factor, inflammation is an imbedded mechanism of developed cardiovascular diseases including coagulation, atherosclerosis, metabolic syndrome, insulin resistance, and diabetes mellitus," says a 2017 study[7]. "It is also associated with development of non-cardiovascular diseases such as psoriasis, depression, cancer, and renal [kidney] diseases."
- **Seventy to eighty percent of your immune system lies in your gut,** states this 2008 study[8]. It's there to tell if what you've swallowed is friend or foe, and to react against what's not good for you with inflammation.
- **Obesity raises infection and death risk,** found this 2011 study[9] on Influenza (H1N1) pandemic in California. Fifty-one percent of patients hospitalized were obese (BMI > 30), and 19% were extremely obese (BMI > 40). Among the deaths, "61% were obese and 30% were extremely obese."

Next, impaired mouth Structure contributes to obstructive sleep apnea (OSA) and leading killer diseases as follows:

- "OSA brings many adverse consequences, such as hypertension, obesity, diabetes mellitus, cardiac and encephalic [brain] alterations, behavioral, among others," says this 2016 study[10].
- "Sleep apnea (SA) is linked to a variety of disorders, particularly cardiovascular diseases," concludes this 2017 study[11]. It found SA patients have 11 times the risk of death with co-existent conditions like respiratory infection or diabetes compared to those without.
- This 2019 study[12] states, "OSA patients show a high prevalence of:
  - cardiovascular diseases: systemic hypertension, coronary artery disease, arrhythmias, ischemic stroke,
  - respiratory diseases COPD, asthma, and
  - metabolic disorders (diabetes mellitus, dyslipidemia, gout)."

Higher susceptibility to killer diseases comes from a combination of Impaired Mouth Syndrome and an impaired mouth style. Helping your health thrive starts with Holistic Mouth Solutions to support sleep without airway obstruction and sensible eating without fueling inflammation.

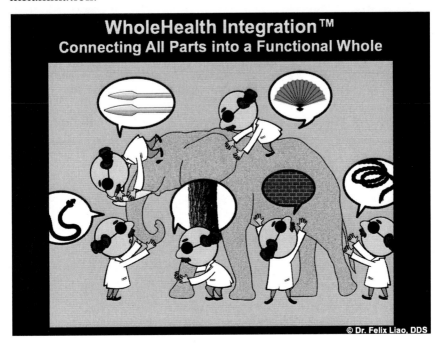

Big-Picture Questions

Can you put my body back together so my health works for me again? That's an unspoken question many of my new patients have. They are tired of the usual Band-Aid approach and side effects. Managing symptoms with drugs, surgery, drills, and night guards has not solved their problems. Like Helen earlier, they've "circled the blocks" many times already. Not always spoken, but nonetheless on their minds: "What'll happen to me next? Can I be well again?"

Deep sleep from good mouth Structure and knowing how to eat for health (smarter mouth Style) are increasingly important as you age from 30s into 50s and beyond. As the owner of your health, your job is to provide your body with:

1. Sound teeth free of jaw infections to provide stem cells (from around their roots) to restart impaired mouth Structure development to widen airway.
2. An airway-centered checkup of your mouth Structure to determine whether it's a health asset or a liability.
3. A low-inflammation diet and bone-building eating Style to regrow your jaws and renew all parts of your body.

Low energy, high blood pressure/sugar, heavier weight, and worn-down teeth are warning lights on your dashboard. How should you respond as the operator of your mouth?

The U-Turn Back Toward Thriving Health & Wellness

1. **Impaired Mouth Syndrome diagnosis by AMD + Sleep Test as needed;**

2. **Clean up mouth infections: infected root canals, jaw cavitations, bleeding gums;**

3. **Redevelop "3-Foot Cage" with epigenetic oral sleep appliances;**

4. **Check & fix adrenals + thyroids + vitamin D + B;**

5. **Restore deep and refreshing sleep;**

6. **Restore nasal breathing; ID food sensitivity and eliminate nasal obstruction;**

7. **Adopt Holistic Mouth Style: healthier diet and sensible eating.**

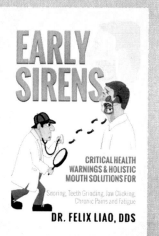

EARLY SIRENS

CRITICAL HEALTH WARNINGS & HOLISTIC MOUTH SOLUTIONS FOR

Snoring, Teeth Grinding, Jaw Clicking, Chronic Pains and Fatigue

DR. FELIX LIAO, DDS

Your whole body pays a huge price if your mouth is structurally impaired and/or overused. Many symptoms (pain and fatigue) and conditions (inflammation and obesity) resolve fully or partially when your mouth Structure and Style are aligned with sound health-keeping principles.

WholeHealth Integration

- Cancer can kill, so can sleep apnea, so can inflammation-initiated heart disease, diabetes—*all* have major contributions from both mouth Structure and Style.

- Your impaired mouth Style is the source of gut inflammation and obesity, and your impaired mouth Structure is an anatomical source of airway obstruction.

- Keeping and recovering your health starts with Holistic Mouth Solutions to support sleep without airway obstruction and sensible eating without fueling inflammation. Both mouth Style and Structure are crucial to your whole-body health. If you've already covered one, then work on the other.

Chapter 2

How Holistic Mouth Solutions Work: 3 Case Studies

"Overweight/obesity is a common, reversible risk factor for obstructive sleep apnea severity."

~ American Thoracic Society 2018 Official Clinical Practice Guidelines[1]

A Holistic Mouth is structurally fit to support whole-body health through Alignment, Breathing, Circulation, Digestion, Energy, and Sleep (ABCDES). "Structurally fit" means fully developed jaws, with room for all 32 natural teeth to line up straight naturally in the absence of health disruptors. With fully developed jaws come a wide-open airway to support sleep and provide all the oxygen needed.

A Holistic Mouth Structure by itself can be a solution to many chronic pain conditions in simple cases, as shown in *Early Sirens* and *6-Foot Tiger 3-Foot Cage*. Holistic Mouth Solutions are the combination of necessary Structure and Style to support ABCDES with functional airway and sensible nutrition. Holistic Mouth Solutions can be the start or part of a multi-prong solution in complex cases.

Most chronic diseases are multi-causal: genes, lifestyle, gender, diet, socio-economics, stress, sleep, and now jaws and mouth. The same with sleep apnea and Impaired Mouth Syndrome.

"Obesity and particularly central adiposity are potent risk factors for sleep apnea," states this 2008 study[2]. Keep this point in mind as we see how health's downhill slide and recovery start with the mouth through the cases of Jenna, Joey, and Lucy.

Jenna's Traumatic Injury: Recovery Started with Dr. Liao's Start Thriving Appliance™

Jenna, age 37 and a mother of 3, came to me after having seen 25 doctors in the previous 12 months following a traumatic injury to the base of her head at work. Her presenting symptoms included: dizziness, difficulty falling asleep and staying asleep, snoring, sound and light sensitivity, and various types of headaches including migraine. She also could not perform basic daily tasks, and at times could not speak or find her memory after her injury, sometimes even wheelchair-bound. She could barely walk with the assistance of a cane when I first met her.

In my evaluation, I found that her leg length was uneven because her upper and lower dental midlines were off, as shown in the next slide. Her leg length became even when I gave her a simple stick to bite on between her front teeth, and her dental midlines matched up without her knowing. In addition, she could walk with far greater ease and steadiness right away—it was as if her neurological system came back to life.

Jenna's structurally impaired mouth was interfering with her recovery. I converted that trial bite into a simple upper Start Thriving Appliance™ to free her brain from the tyranny of her structurally impaired mouth. "I was highly skeptical at first," she said. "Now that's all gone, along with my inability to walk, find words and live a normal life." You can see videos of Jenna's remarkable one-month and two-year follow-ups here[3].

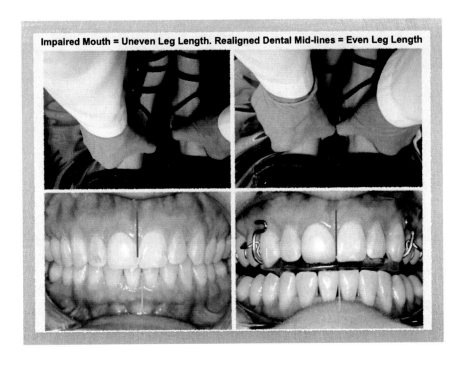

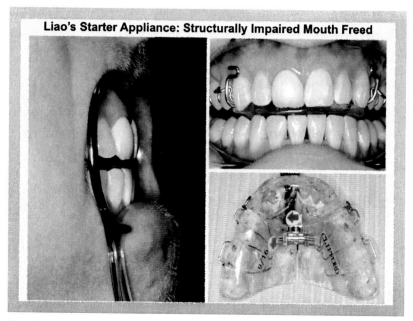

Liao's Starter Appliance: Structurally Impaired Mouth Freed

Dr. Liao's Start Thriving Appliance™ starts the recovery from Impaired Mouth Syndrome by freeing the body from the tyranny of the "6-foot tiger" (oversized tongue) choking the airway because of the "3-foot cage" (underdeveloped jaws).

How was that possible? First, Jenna was a compliant "top-tier" patient who put all my advice into practice. Partial compliance means lesser success. Secondly, Dr. Liao's Start Thriving Appliance™ (STA) helped her sleep and breathe better to start her healing. STA provides a simple "test drive" to see how much Impaired Mouth Syndrome interferes with your life. It has flexible features built-in to treat further—after a favorable "test drive."

The Earth is longer flat in dentistry, and jaw-airway-facial redevelopment is a new frontier in healthcare with the advent of Holistic Mouth Solutions.

Epigenetic Oral Appliance for Adults

Epigenetics is a revolutionary concept from the Human Genome Project for actualizing full genetic potential in the dental-facial development of children and adults alike, regardless of age.

Epi- is a Greek prefix meaning on top of, or in addition to. So, epigenetics refers to factors that overlay your genes and their expression. Nutrition is one epigenetic factor—so is lifestyle, mouth breathing, and certain types of oral appliances. Growth hormone is released in deep sleep in the absence of airway obstruction. The science of stem cell activation with epigenetic oral appliance can be found in chapter 16 of *6-Foot Tiger 3-Foot Cage*.

Dr. Ted Belfor[4] defines epigenetic orthopedics as *"light cyclical forces* provided by removable oral appliances to activate various genes encoded for craniofacial symmetry, tooth straightening, new bone and cartilage growth."

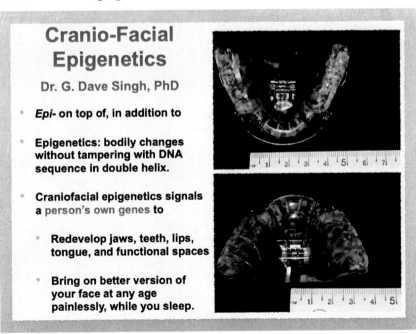

The Daytime and Nighttime (DNA, aka biomimetic) appliance pictured above is developed by Dr. G. Dave Singh, my mentor and inspiration.

In my experience, an epigenetic oral appliance (EOA) can bring out a better version of your face, jaws, and upper airway painlessly while you sleep. Properly designed and used, EOA activates your own genes (so you are still 100% you) to redevelop deficient jaws to your full genetic potential, with room for all your teeth to line up straight naturally. Sometimes, braces or clear aligners are needed to finish.

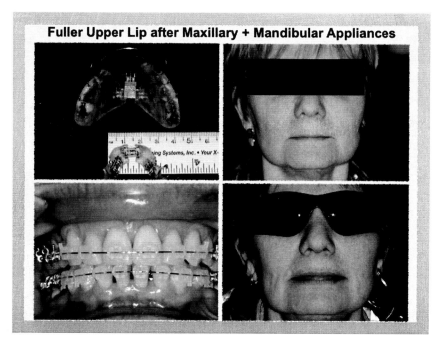

Fuller Upper Lip after Maxillary + Mandibular Appliances

EOAs can redevelop both maxilla and mandible and improve facial appearance, while a mandibular advancement device (MAD) cannot. EOAs can also widen the "three-foot cage" and thereby widen a narrow airway. This is a true root-cause solution.

"Sixty-four percent decrease in AHI [sleep test score]" was reported by this 2016 study[5], which concluded, "Biomimetic oral appliance therapy may be a useful method of managing severe cases of OSA in adults, and represents an alternative to CPAP and MADs."

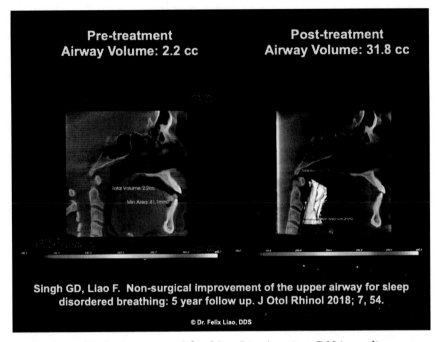

Pre-treatment
Airway Volume: 2.2 cc

Post-treatment
Airway Volume: 31.8 cc

Singh GD, Liao F. Non-surgical improvement of the upper airway for sleep disordered breathing: 5 year follow up. J Otol Rhinol 2018; 7, 54.

© Dr. Felix Liao, DDS

Above: published case study[6] of Dr. Liao's using DNA appliance to redevelop an extremely narrow airway from 2.2 cc (all black going off the color scale) to 31.8 cc (all white) non-surgically.

Better yet, as Kim's and Miss Miller's cases have shown, EOAs can correct chronic neck-shoulder-back pain by redeveloping deficient upper jaw enough for the lower jaw to fit like a foot into a shoe without strain without drilling, shots, surgery, or drugs. In addition to deeper sleep and fixing pain, EOA can also lead to facial glow, fuller lips, nasal breathing, and more—see chapter 4. Can your night guard or MAD do all that?

The Case of Joey

Next comes Joey, a 52-year-old executive newly referred by his hormone doctor. He had Obstructive Sleep Apnea (OSA), disliked his CPAP mask, and wanted a more root-cause solution.

Jenna and Joey both suffer from Impaired Mouth Syndrome, but their treatment will be vastly different. Joey has a pot belly and a bulge under his lower jaw from ear to ear: "I am now 310 pounds, and my goal is 240 for my 6-foot-2 frame." Not surprisingly, he has low back pain, snores, and grinds his teeth, and his airway is 80% occupied by his tongue.

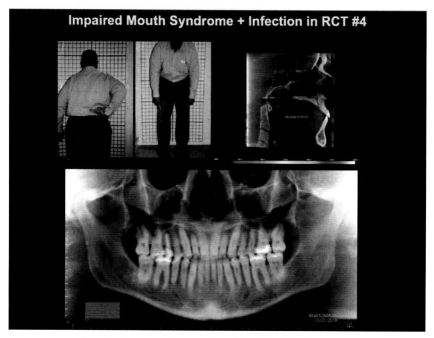

Joey's airway is beyond red (in the black zone)—
imagine having an angel-hair pasta for his oxygen pipeline.

Joey's airway was occupied by an "eight-foot tiger"—an oversized tongue (due to his excess weight)—forced into his throat because it doesn't fit in his "three-foot cage." No mechanical device or appliance will ever be its match.

Dentally, Joey had perfectly clean teeth, no cavities, no gum disease. However, Joey's CT scan shows a dark shadow at the end of a root-canaled tooth suggestive of infection and cardiovascular risk.

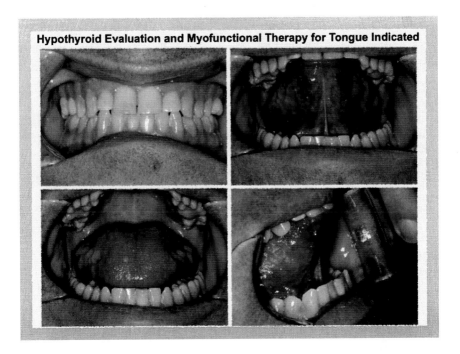

Hypothyroid Evaluation and Myofunctional Therapy for Tongue Indicated

Seen through a mouth doctor's eyes, Joey's tongue appears swollen and suggestive of hypothyroidism (low thyroid), which can contribute to his overweight and airway struggles. The scalloped borders of his tongue are 70% specific for sleep apnea, as reported by this 2005 study[7].

Joey's airway treatment needs more WholeHealth Integration, including hormonal evaluation (and support), PLUS mouth Style reform—how much he eats, how often, at what speed, how long before sleep, not just what he eats. As he said, "My job includes lots of client entertainment and eating out. I know all too well my weight is a problem because my knees hurt when I walk."

"Weight-loss interventions, especially comprehensive lifestyle interventions, are associated with improvements in OSA severity, cardio-metabolic co-morbidities, and quality of life," states American Thoracic Society[8]. It "recommends that clinicians regularly assess weight and incorporate weight management strategies that are tailored to individual patient preferences into the routine treatment of adult patients with OSA who are overweight or obese."

Whether Joey sticks with his CPAP mask or starts oral appliance to widen his airway, adopting a holistic mouth Style on how to eat is critical for his wellness and immunity.

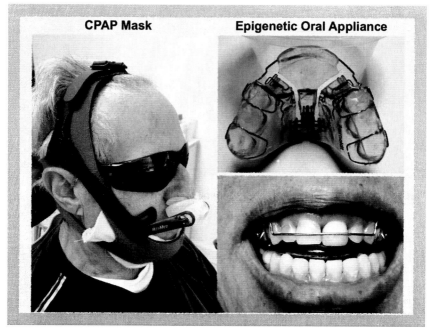

CPAP mask and epigenetic oral appliance have different indications, plusses, and minuses. Talk to your sleep doctor or Airway-centered Mouth Doctor about [American Academy of Sleep Medicine Guideline for Oral Appliances (2015)][9].

WholeHealth Alignment with Your Healthcare Professionals

Obesity, sleep apnea, heart disease, and cancer are outcomes. What are the causes, and does your healthcare address them? This has everything to do with your life quality and healthcare cost.

When you see your healthcare professionals (HCPs), is the focus on symptom management or root-cause solutions? Is your relationship based on medications for this symptom, an operation for that problem, or insurance coverage? This is an individual decision driven by personal values and life circumstances.

Does your "health insurance" coverage come with side effects? What if it offers "Band-Aids" and not root-cause solutions? Do you go with its "coverage" or go "out of network" to pay for what's best for your health? The road also forks here.

If root-cause solutions matter more to you, then consider looking for root-cause oriented HCPs. Pay out of your own pocket for proactive coaching. Pennies spent this way can save you tons of trouble later. I'm most fortunate to have found these professionals to support me on my own journey:

- An acupuncturist with the smarts of a lawyer and the heart of an angel. She'd offer her own lunch if my patients showed up for their first visit without breakfast or lunch: "You need to have enough energy to respond well to treatment." That's on top of being well-versed in East-West nutrition and the keenest diagnostician I know. She'd call me out with one glance, "Did you stay up late again?"

- A surgeon turned integrative hormone doctor as my medical mentor. He has treated urinary tract infections with diet and added probiotics, and men with erectile dysfunction with not just a pill, but attention to all blood vessels at risk, including oral contribution to sleep apnea. That's only one indication of his root-cause digging. He travels the world to seek out the best digestive formula for dense breast disease, prostate enlargement, and wellness maintenance alike. His liquid oxygen supplement can support fatigue, brain fog, diabetic ulcers, and more.

- An Airway-centered Mouth Doctor® and biological dentist who knows how to integrate everything described in this book with respect to implant surgery. Every detail is included—from vitamin D to antioxidants before surgery and lymph drainage afterward, to lodging at a B&B with an angelic hostess and door-to-door service.

- A dermatologist who didn't just give me steroid creams for my "allergic reaction" to latex gloves. She dug deep into the root causes and treated me from the inside out. That's how I learned about adrenal depletion and toxic burdens, and how to work my way back from "running on fumes."

These health-builders and I have a patient-doctor relationship that is not bound by insurance terms. We agree to focus on treating the root causes of my symptoms. I learn something healthful and helpful from each visit, and I'm better off after doing what they say. This WholeHealth alignment provided me the energy and health to write this book, and to bring greater success to cases like Lucy's.

Lucy's Case: Breakthrough Outcome from WholeHealth Integration

Lucy had come from Hawaii to see me in metro DC after reading my first two books. Her complaints included neck and shoulder pain, daytime sleepiness, tingling and numbness in both feet, and a lifetime of being 40 pounds overweight.

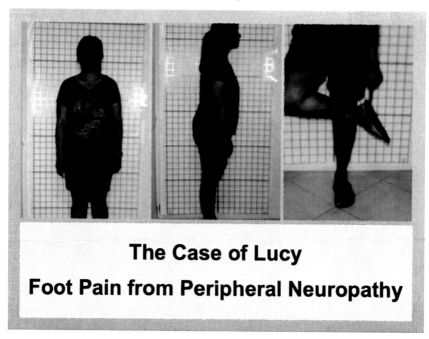

The Case of Lucy
Foot Pain from Peripheral Neuropathy

I did my diagnostic workup and referred her to my acupuncturist, who coached her on best lifestyle practices: diaphragm (belly) breathing, how to stand and walk (ditch the flip flops), and what to eat for her constitution type. I also sent her to my MD for thyroid and hormonal support for sleep. Lucy went home with his advice on a ketogenic diet along with an individualized appliance.

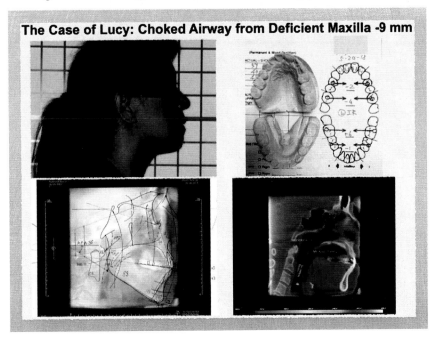

The Case of Lucy: Choked Airway from Deficient Maxilla -9 mm

Lucy took this WholeHealth Integration to heart and did it faithfully upon returning home. She has since lost 60 pounds and now fits into the dresses of her college-age daughters. (Lucy's husband went along with her new eating style, too, and his back pain went from major debilitation to minor annoyance after losing 50 pounds.)

Lucy is loving her newfound energy after stopping all added sugars and carbs and eating nothing processed: "Stopping nightshades [potatoes, tomatoes, bell peppers] and taking up intermittent fasting made a dramatic difference." (That does not mean you need to stop eating nightshades vegetables. Consult with your HCP if you have non-resolving inflammation, or type "nightshades and inflammation" into your search engine for more information.)

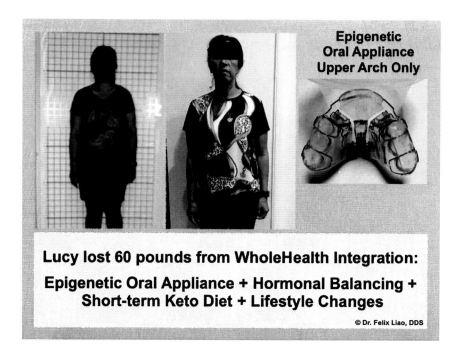

Epigenetic Oral Appliance Upper Arch Only

Lucy lost 60 pounds from WholeHealth Integration:

Epigenetic Oral Appliance + Hormonal Balancing + Short-term Keto Diet + Lifestyle Changes

© Dr. Felix Liao, DDS

Eighteen months after starting her oral appliance, Lucy's progress includes:

- Neuropathy symptoms dropping from 10 to 6 on a 10-point scale.
- Arthritis symptoms dropping from 5.5 to 0, and medications stopped.
- Systolic blood pressure dropping 20 mm Hg, from 130-140 to 110-120.
- Improved sleep: she wakes up ahead of her alarm clock, feeling refreshed.

Such results take a WholeHealth team with aligned values *and* a compliant patient who puts both the advice and device into practice.

"Keep doing what you are doing, and don't come back," Lucy's rheumatologist said to her six months after starting this airway-centered WholeHealth Integration. Although Lucy's case is still in progress, it's fair to say that her health and quality of life in the next decade will be far superior than the previous.

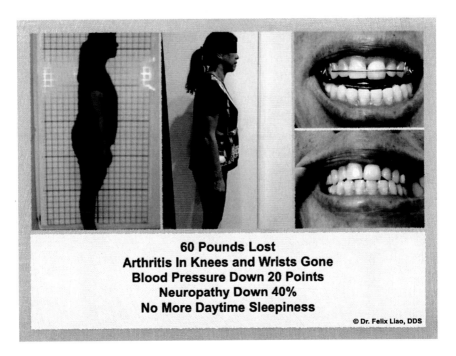

60 Pounds Lost
Arthritis In Knees and Wrists Gone
Blood Pressure Down 20 Points
Neuropathy Down 40%
No More Daytime Sleepiness

© Dr. Felix Liao, DDS

By teaching patients how to brush and floss, the dental profession created a paradigm shift from extracting diseased teeth to preserving natural teeth for life. Can redeveloping their "3-foot cage" and getting them "licensed to thrive" do the same to save more hearts, brains, breasts, prostates, and joints at much lower costs than usual? I believe the answer is yes.

WholeHealth Integration

- How did Jenna, Joey, and Lucy arrive at their symptoms and wilted state of health? The mouth had been missing in all their visits to their own dentists and healthcare professionals (HCPs).

- Sleep and oxygen are not optional in keeping or recovering your health. Combining holistic mouth Structure and Style with WholeHealth Integration can deliver breakthrough results.

- The next step is for healthcare professionals to recognize the impact of Impaired Mouth Syndrome and Holistic Mouth Solutions on their patients' health: *What does it take to restore every patient into a functional and sustainable Whole?*

Chapter 3

Inflammation, Infections, and Your Mouth

"Inflammation is the major driver of human disease. It damages your heart, your brain, your kidneys, your gut. Poor-quality sleep, especially sleep apnea, creates a persistent inflammatory state in your body."

~ Cecilia Wu, M.D.,
Anatomic, Forensic, and Cardiovascular Pathologist

Epigenetic oral appliance therapy can help redevelop deficient jaws and narrow airway to deliver oxygen, mitigate pain, and promote sleep. But there's a pre-condition: Your mouth must be free of dental infections and gum inflammation.

Inflammation is the body's response to an injury in the interest of survival and renewal. A carpet burn or scrape on your knee will be red, hot, throbbing, and painful. Those are all signs of inflammation, the start of the process to heal.

That same kind of burn or inflammation can happen on the inside of your body and arteries, too, in response to dental infections[1] or ingestion of sugary foods[2]. The lining of your circulatory system is only one cell thick, just like that of your gut and gums, and thus susceptible to injury and infection.

All parts of the body are interconnected, but America's healthcare remains a fragmented piece-meal. Biological dentists[3] do more than just drill and fill teeth; biological dentists see to it that your mouth is a health asset rather than a liability.

"Oral health is more than healthy teeth"—it's time for all dentists to put this point from the U.S. Surgeon General[4] into patient care. It's also time for all healthcare professionals to know how sleep apnea-driven inflammation and chronic pain rooted in impaired mouth Structure can be greatly mitigated or resolved by collaborating with an Airway-centered Mouth Doctor (AMD).

From the Mouth to Whole-Body Health Troubles

Widespread ignorance of oral contributions to medical symptoms can have serious consequences. In 2030, cancer will kill twice as many people as in 1968.

"When I started my cancer clinic 20 years ago, the average age of my patients was 60. Today, it's 30," said Dr. Antonio Jimenez, MD, author of *HopeForCancer*. Speaking on "Dental Toxins in Integrative Cancer Therapy" in the 2019 Annual Meeting of iabdm. org, Dr. Jimenez is among a small but growing number of doctors who get the imperative necessity of biological dentistry. His cancer clinic has seen 70% more new cases. Why?

"Local problems don't stay local," Dr. Jimenez said. "Cancer is not just local [be it breast or colon], but systemic dysregulation. Inflammation fuels tumor growth and metastasis."

That last line jumped out at me. Combine Dr. Jimenez's statement with Dr. Wu's at the top, you can see that cancer control starts with inflammation control. Ditto all degenerative diseases.

If limiting inflammation is critical, then your mouth is where you want to take charge. How? Start with making sure your mouth is free from toxins and infections with a biological dentist. Then, have your mouth Structure checked by a qualified mouth doctor and adopt a holistic mouth Style to limit oral contribution to internal inflammation.

Indeed, the mouth plays a role in 6 of Dr. Jimenez's "7 Keys of Integrative Cancer Therapy": immune modulation, full-spectrum nutrition, detoxification, oxygenation, restoration of the microbiome, and spiritual and emotional healing.

Your body has a set of basic needs. Seeing to those needs is your job as the owner of your health. First and foremost: airway rules. Oxygen is not optional, nor is sleep. With mouth structure un-impaired, plus wholesome foods, clean air, and water, your body can run itself. In biological medicine and dentistry, this is called self-regulation.

Dysregulation is what happens when your body lacks what it needs to fight toxins and infections over time. You then become susceptible to fatigue, infections, inflammation, illness, and premature death. Autoimmune disorders are dysregulation gone wild, and the immune system has turned against the body it's meant to protect, as in rheumatoid arthritis and Hashimoto's thyroiditis.

The Oral Origin of Heart Disease and Other Killer Diseases

Heart disease is the leading cause of death in first-world countries, and it starts in the mouth. Diet plays a role. So does stress, sleep, and airway obstruction.

Science now says heart disease stems from inflammation's cumulative damages inside artery walls. "Most researchers agree that atherosclerosis starts as an inflammation," writes Dr. Uffe

Ravnskov in his brilliant book *Ignore the Awkward*, in which he debunks the cholesterol myth. Among his key points are:

- "There is also general agreement that atherosclerosis, heart disease and stroke are associated in some way with infectious diseases."

- "Mental stress, another established risk factor, stimulates production of the hormone cortisol, and an excess of cortisol promotes infections."

- Eliminating chronic oral infections helps: "Dental researchers from Italy for instance treated 35 otherwise healthy individuals with evidence of periodontal infections. After the treatment, examination of the carotid arterial wall showed that its thickness had diminished significantly and much more than seen in any cholesterol-lowering trial."

- A good amount of evidence actually suggests that inflammation of the arteries isn't the main cause of heart problems. Rather, inflammation is "a secondary phenomenon caused by microorganisms or their toxins." [This harks back to his first point on infection.]

- It's not just the germs, but the factors that support them: "It is not the water that causes the boat to go down; it is the iceberg that staved in the keel."

Cholesterol isn't the start of heart disease, though this notion will die hard in some minds. Dr. Ravnskov is hardly a lone maverick on the infectious origin of cardiovascular disease.

The circulatory system within a tooth's root canals is as complex as the cardiovascular tree—see for yourself by typing "root canal anatomy by Professor Walter Hess" into your search engine. Once the nerve and other tissues inside a tooth are dead, the spider webs and catacomb spaces (imagine an English muffin or cinder block) offer a perfect haven for bugs to stay beyond the reach of immune cells and antibiotics. This is one reason why many patients complain that some root-canaled teeth "never quite feel right." Root canal anatomy makes it an impossibly tall order for treatment to be 100% successful.

A root-canaled tooth is a dead tooth. "Loss of circulation to the dental organ leaves a 'gangrenous tissue,'" says Dr. Ronald Carlson, DDS, author of *Death by Root Canal*[6]. Dr. Carlson writes regarding the 364 reports on over 400 extracted root-canaled teeth by board-certified pathologists from Hawaii's Queen's Hospital, "In most every case there was an inflammatory, infected, or degenerate condition (reactive bone lesions), often with *actinomycotic* organisms observed 45—50% of the time."

Loss of circulation means more bacterial/fungal/viral infections due to loss of local immunity. This common sense is born out in the following selective studies.

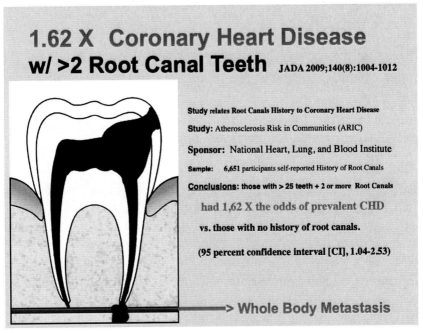

1.62 X Coronary Heart Disease
w/ >2 Root Canal Teeth   JADA 2009;140(8):1004-1012

Study relates Root Canals History to Coronary Heart Disease

Study: Atherosclerosis Risk in Communities (ARIC)

Sponsor: National Heart, Lung, and Blood Institute

Sample: 6,651 participants self-reported History of Root Canals

Conclusions: those with > 25 teeth + 2 or more Root Canals

had 1.62 X the odds of prevalent CHD

vs. those with no history of root canals.

(95 percent confidence interval [CI], 1.04-2.53)

—> Whole Body Metastasis

This 2009 study[7] shows that people with 2 or more root-canaled teeth have a 62% higher risk for coronary heart disease.

Viruses are found in 18 of 21 studies in this 2016 review[8] of studies on the virus-root canal disease link: "The main association between viruses and endodontic pathosis [root-canals related disease] is between Cytomegalovirus and Epstein-Barr [EB] virus." The EB virus had a 41% presence in the studies compared to 2% in controls.

Dr. Thomas E. Levy, MD, is another enlightened cardiologist who includes the mouth as a prime suspect in heart disease, cancer, and other killers. The subtitle of his book *Hidden Epidemics*[9] speaks volumes: *Silent Oral Infections Cause Most Heart Attacks and Breast Cancers*. This landmark work reunites dentistry with medicine and links infectious and environmental toxins with the chronic degenerative diseases killing most Americans today.

Some doctors will balk at accepting the infectious origin of heart disease, much like those in 1982 when Drs. Barry Marshall and Robin Warren suggested that the bacterium *H. pylori* was the cause of stomach ulcers. Yet this is common knowledge today.

H. pylori infection has since been linked to stomach cancer and duodenal ulcers as well. Eighty percent of those infected with it have no symptoms. *H. pylori* has been found in saliva and dental plaque, as well as feces. Marshall and Warren were awarded the Nobel Prize in Medicine in 2005 for their work in this area.

The idea that oral infections can cause distant health problems is hardly far-fetched. Opening a closed mind can be awkward, but with such ignorance and resistance comes a high cost: continued suffering and possibly premature death.

This is not to say I am against root-canal treatment across the board. When my son had a lacrosse accident at age 15, I did a root canal for his damaged upper front tooth but let him know the risks. He's now 38 and a father himself. I continue to keep my eyes on his tooth and total health.

When considering root canal treatment, I do feel it's wise to assess each patient's overall health, medical dental history, and systemic fitness to handle the infection from one more dead tooth—in consultation with your attending doctors and dentists. That's particularly important in immune-compromised patients with cancer, diabetes, and heart and neuro-degenerative diseases.

"Practically all chronic diseases originate in the gut, including cavities and periodontal disease," writes Dr. Alvin Danenberg, an integrative periodontist and author of *Is Your Gut Killing You?*[10] "The mouth may be a toxic time bomb. Most people, including medical and dental professionals, don't realize the enormous consequences."

Cavitational Osteonecrosis - also known as jaw "cavitations," these are another oral source of toxins that can undermine health. *Osteo-* means bone; *-necrosis* means death.

Cavitations (cavities in the jaw) are typically extraction sites with diseased or dead bone. Healthy bone is moist and bleeds red and freely when surgically opened, whereas a cavitation oozes tar-like black sludge. Some cavitation can be a dry rot that does not bleed (ie., lifeless). A biopsy is a simple way to tell.

"While still little recognized or even appreciated by mainstream dentistry," writes Dr. Levy in *Hidden Epidemics*[11], "it is nevertheless an extremely prevalent condition. Cavitations were clearly present in at least 88% (313 of 354 sites) explored in 112 randomly selected patients."

Eighty-eight percent! For most of my dentist colleagues, this is too hard to swallow—just as it was for many doctors to believe *H. pylori* could cause ulcers earlier. Yet should we dismiss it lightly? Is it more important to save a tooth, or a heart and a life?

My Own Case Story

I had my wisdom teeth extracted in dental school as a student. I had discovered cavitations in those sites 15 years ago, but I didn't do anything about them. After all, I felt healthy and vigorous. I didn't have any symptoms...until about a year ago. Inexplicably, I began to have a series of troubles: painfully swollen ankles (first left, then right), blisters erupting between my fingers in both hands, and two dead lower first molars—the ones that do all the chewing and bring pleasure to eating. It was time to respond to my body's messages.

I chose Dr. Judson Wall—a biological dentist in Bountiful, Utah—to clean out my jaw cavitations. After a world-class diagnostic process, we put together a pre-op protocol that included two months of IV chelation therapy to remove both environmental and internal toxins, and to boost my vitamin D, antioxidants, and adrenals.

We also did a heart rate variability (HRV) test before the surgery and one day after. HRV measures physical fitness and adaptive reserve, with a score of 1/1 (top left corner) being peak fitness and 13/7 total system collapse. Here's how my results looked, with the blue arrow in the right panel showing the amount of improvement:

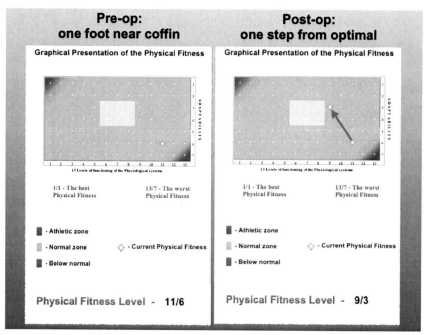

As the blue arrow shows in the right image, I went from having one foot in the coffin at 11/6 to near normal at 9/3 just one day after jaw cavitation surgery.

As you can see, the cavitations were a huge deal to my overall health. The body can heal itself once you get the thorn out—jaw cavitation in this case.

Do you have oral contributions to chronic inflammation and systemic symptoms? See a qualified biological dentist.

Got Impaired Mouth Syndrome? See an Airway-centered Mouth Doctor®.

WholeHealth Integration

- Biologically sound teeth and gums are the foundation to redevelop deficient jaws with epigenetic oral appliances to widen airway and deepen sleep.

- No sound teeth, no epigenetic solution. Make sure your teeth, gums, and jaws are free of infection and inflammation.

- I encourage wellness-minded dentists to become biological dentists (iabdm.org). After all, what good is having the best-looking set of teeth in the morgue?

- A holistic mouth Structure and Style combine to lower inflammation and promote immunity through deep sleep.

Chapter 4

Your Digestive System and Gut Microbiome

"In the intestines lies Life, or Death."

~ Dietrich Klinghardt, MD, PhD

Life is a treat when your digestion works. Life is hell when it doesn't—just ask anyone with constipation or irritable bowel. The difference comes largely from your mouth Style, or how you use your mouth.

At the smell of baked goods or grilled meats, saliva starts to flow. You take a bite. The texture of the food, the chewing, the mixing of saliva with the food, the taste…these not only give you oral pleasure; they simultaneously signal to your gut what's coming. Seamless coordination is how your digestion is designed to work.

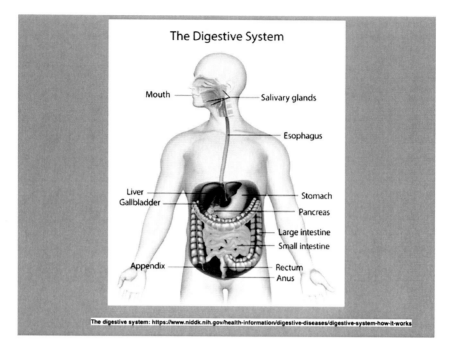

The digestive system: https://www.niddk.nih.gov/health-information/digestive-diseases/digestive-system-how-it-works

Your digestive system's job is to make energy by extracting nutrients from food and drink through a top-down sequence:

- Ingestion, in the mouth
- Digestion, in the stomach
- Absorption, in the small intestine (gut)
- Immune defense, in the gut
- Microbiome symbiosis, in the colon
- Waste elimination (mild) and toxins rejection (strong)

Ingestion in the 2020s: First-World Countries

"Overeating must be understood as part of the wider cultural problem of consumption and materialism," writes Kim Cargill in *The Psychology of Overeating*[1].

Why do TV commercials, billboards, and pop-up ads push foods in your face all the time? As Michael Moss reported in his superb book *Salt, Sugar, Fat: How Food Giants Hooked Us*[2]:

"Every year, the average American eats thirty-three pounds of cheese and seventy pounds of sugar. Every day, we ingest eighty-five hundred milligrams of salt, double the recommended amount, almost none of which comes from the shakers on our table."

Your body is not designed to handle that much year after year. "Oh, but it tastes great!" The slick commercials and shiny packages are designed to make you salivate like Pavlov's dogs, and they succeed all too well. With over-consumption comes a serious health consequence to the one-cell-thick lining of your gut and arterial tree.

Americans are awash in a sea of cheap, hyper-processed, factory-prepared foods. We are targeted with "techniques taken straight from the Big Tobacco playbook," writes Moss.

"It's cheap, attractive and convenient, and we eat it every day—it's difficult not to. But is ultra-processed food making us ill and driving the global obesity crisis?" Bee Wilson asks in her article in The Guardian[3] with a spot-on title: *How Ultra-Processed Food Took Over Your Shopping Basket.*

Indigestion and Inflammation

When you go out to eat in a typical American restaurant, the first thing you're given is usually ice water, followed perhaps with bread and butter. This is such a pervasive cultural norm that no one stops to consider its health implications.

By contrast, you're served hot tea when you go to an authentic Chinese restaurant. There's a good reason: warmer food temperature means better digestion. Putting a drink 60 degrees colder than your body temperature into your stomach retards digestion. That sets the stage for gut inflammation, which can result in these signs and symptoms:

- "Love handles," a.k.a. central obesity—there's nothing cute about it medically

- Metabolic syndrome, diabetes, high blood pressure, peripheral neuropathy, obstructive sleep apnea, hypothyroidism, and more
- Bloating, heartburn, acid reflux, gas, burping, constipation, diarrhea, and other abdominal disease or discomfort
- Nasal congestion, sinusitis, postnasal drip, coughing, throat tickles
- Fatigue, lack of motivation, brain fog
- Tingling, itching, eczema, blisters, hives, and other skin issues
- Swollen tongue, coated tongue, tooth prints on the sides of the tongue
- Muscle pain in the neck, shoulder, back, and/or jaw
- Reduced immunity to infections, cancer, heart disease, and more
- Stress-related symptoms, including fatigue, insomnia, depression, anxiety

And that's just a partial list! How do you respond? Go to the doctor(s), drug store, emergency, or operating room? How about changing your mouth Style instead? It's time to train the owner-operator with the equivalent of "driver's education."

Congestion and "Leaky Gut"

Congestion comes from both overfeeding and intestinal (gut) inflammation. The primitive brain is programmed to reject rotten or bitter food and to like crunchy, tangy, and sweet-tasting foods. It's only human to want more of what's "tasty," and that's where we get manipulated by food manufacturers. "I dare you to eat just one" is both a dare and a mock. One result of runaway consumption to satisfy "taste" is congestion.

Once you swallow that tasty steak, chicken, burger, pizza, or soda, your digestive tract is tasked with dealing with it, attempting to break down the protein with stomach acids. The efficiency of this critical digestive stage is cut down by ice water, age, stress, excess salt, added sugars, trans fats, etc.

With incompletely digested protein comes inflammation leading to leaky gut, the common name for increased intestinal permeability. Leaky gut opens the door to multiple sensitivities, food intolerances, and autoimmune dysregulation, including rheumatoid arthritis, gluten sensitivity, irritable bowel syndrome, and more.

Recall that inflammation is the body's response to something that it either rejects or needs to recover from. "Before chronic disease, there is inflammation, but before inflammation comes gut dysfunction. Anti-inflammation treatment helps, but gut repair corrects the problem right at its source," writes Dr. Alejandro Junger in *Clean Gut*[4]. With his kind permission, here are some highlights.

> "When I use the word gut, however, I refer to a lot more than just the body's digestive tube. I mean the living organisms inside the gut, the intestinal flora, and the immune and nervous systems within and around the walls of the intestines. The body doesn't make a distinction between these different parts. Nor should we."

Most of us are born with an intact and fully capable digestive system. Oral infections and gut inflammation are either human-made or self-induced by impaired mouth Style. "We are all walking around with damaged guts and, to different degrees, suffering the consequences in day-to-day and long-term health," adds Dr. Junger.

> "Without an optimally functioning gut, we simply don't have a chance of achieving true long-lasting health. When we repair the gut and eliminate the root of disease, however, major and minor symptoms disappear, and we discover what it means to be truly healthy."

You can eat your way into agonizing illness or thriving wellness. The mouth is where you take control.

The Gut Microbiome in Symbiosis and Dysbiosis

Each of us contains countless microbes—"an abundant microscopic menagerie," as journalist Ed Yong describes it in *I Contain Multitudes*[5]. Collectively, we call them the microbiome:

> "They live inside our bodies ["mostly in the gut"], and sometimes inside our very cells…We can't see any of these minuscule specks. But if our own cells were to mysteriously disappear, they would perhaps be detectable as a ghostly microbial shimmer, outlining a now-vanished animal core. Even when are alone, we are never alone. We exist in symbiosis—a wonderful term that refers to different organisms living together."

Symbiosis works because it's mutually beneficial. The good bacteria help you digest your food, and you feed them with healthy eats. Symbiosis makes synergistic productivity in your gut, health in your body, and a glow on your face.

Dysbiosis results when conditions in the gut favor the growth of bad/harmful bacteria. They take over your gut like rioters terrorizing neighborhoods. Dysbiosis starts inflammation, bloating, and pain in the gut, the brain, and beyond.

Factors favoring dysbiosis include a diet low in fiber but high in sugar and refined carbs (which feed yeasts and cancers alike), medications such as antibiotics and anti-inflammatory steroids, and low oxygen (hypoxia).

Eating a perfect diet isn't enough. Oxygen rules. The mitochondria in our cells make way more energy in the presence of oxygen by processing glucose through what's known as the Krebs cycle[6]. Conversely, oxygen deficiency results in lower energy which favors dysbiosis and diseases. As this 2012 study[7] on cancer proliferation found,

> "Our model represents the first one for explaining what possibly drives cancer growth/accelerated growth…A key inter-

nal driver, that we found, is that the reduced energy efficiency (caused by hypoxia and/or possibly other factors) triggers increased uptake and accumulation of glucose, leading to cell proliferation."

Low oxygen is a trigger for cancer cell proliferation—a potent reminder of why the wide-open airway is so vital. Eating perfectly is not good enough.

Your Health Depends Greatly on Your Gut Microbiome

Your microbiome is a driving force behind the fact that what you eat can affect many common symptoms. "The gut microbiome has also been linked to multiple allergic diseases, including asthma and eczema," notes 2016 Comprehensive Review of the Nasal Microbiome in Chronic Rhinosinusitis[8].

> "It is noteworthy that development of a healthy microbiome in the body is dependent on the individual's exposure to a surrounding environment rich in microbes. Moreover, diversity of microbial exposure is inversely correlated with development of allergic and inflammatory conditions such as asthma and allergic rhinitis."

A full discussion of mouth/gut/brain connection is beyond this primer. Nonetheless, I do want you to know this gut-mouth-wellness connection:

> "There is increasing evidence that resident microbial communities in the human gastrointestinal tract, airway, and skin contribute to health and disease. This complex relationship between the microbiota and the human host could lend itself to manipulation to benefit the host."

That comes from The Microbiome in Allergic Disease[9] (2017), which also explains, "Physiological changes, including pH or oxygen level, change the environment…Host-microbe cross-talk is a key determinant of the tissue habitat…which, under steady-state conditions, results in a state of mutualism; however, dysregulation of this interaction, such as through exposure to an exogenous pathogen, medical treatment (antibiotics, antifungal drugs, and immunosuppression), or inflammation/tissue damage, can perpetuate inflammation or cause exacerbation."

Note the roles oxygen, nutrients, diet, and how dysregulation starts in the caption explanation above. Case closed for the crucial roles of Holistic Mouth Structure (oxygen and airway) and Style (diet, lifestyle) in gut health.

Factory Food Additives and Preservatives

There's a clear distinction between farm food and factory food. Farm food is naturally grown from your garden or organic fields responsibly and sustainably run. Factory processed foods come with additives and preserves that can tip the balance inside your gut from symbiosis to dysbiosis.

Simply put, dysbiosis is a depletion of the good bacteria (from antibiotics and anti-inflammatory pills) and an overgrowth of the bad bacteria (from added sugar and food preservatives). "The role of food preservatives as potential triggers of gut microbiota dysbiosis has been long overlooked," states this 2019 study[10]. "To conclude, our data demonstrate that antimicrobial food additives trigger gut microbiota dysbiosis."

Common preservatives include benzoate, sorbate sodium nitrite, calcium propionate, sulphites, and disodium ethylenediaminetetraacetate (EDTA). Here are 22 Food Additives and Preservatives[11].

"The environment created in the gut by ultra-processed foods, a hallmark of the Western diet, is an evolutionarily unique selection ground for microbes that can promote diverse forms of inflammatory disease," notes this 2018 Norway study[12]. "Future research must aim at better identifying which aspects of food processing may impose negative health effects."

Until all the research is completed, what should you do? If thriving health matters to you, then type "Common Food Additives and Preservatives" into your search engine and you'll know the answer. Then, read the next chapter.

WholeHealth Integration

- How well your gut microbiome works as your health partner (in symbiosis) or as your gut terrorists (in dysbiosis) depends on both your mouth Structure *and* Style.

- TV commercials, billboards, and pop-up ads push food in your face all the time? They're designed to make you salivate like Pavlov's dogs.

- To control inflammation, we need to provide "driver's education" to the owner-operator of your mouth to help you stay within guardrails.

- Real foods need no labels: watermelon, salmon, broccoli, potatoes. Factory processed foods come with additives and preservatives. You become what you eat.

Chapter 5

The Good, the Bad, the Terrible

"The only means to fight the plague is honesty."

~ Albert Camus (1947)

Every five days, your gut renews its lining. That's the good news. Given proper care, nutrients, absence of toxins, and oxygen, you can revive your gut in a week in most cases. So, why is gut inflammation such a persistent problem? Answer: toxic health disruptors in modern America.

Health Disruptors

A health disruptor is any substance or condition that interferes with your body's ability to self-regulate. Nails in your car tire or a bent wheel in your bicycle are mechanical disruptors. Similarly, unnatural ingredients ingested can singularly or collectively impair your organ functions: genetically modified organisms (GMOs), food preservatives (to prolong shelf-life of processed foods), food additives (high fructose corn syrup), or plastics from food packaging ending up in wild-caught fish or your baby's cord blood, etc. These are external health disruptors that are in your power to avoid.

Suspect internal health disruptor(s) if your body does not start healing with good sleep and healthy diet in two weeks—that's my rule of thumb based on common sense. Internal health disruptors can include heavy metal toxicity (lead, arsenic, or mercury), medication overdose, undiagnosed conditions such as hypothyroidism, or Impaired Mouth Syndrome. You need a trained healthcare professional to identify and fix them.

The Good

Take a piece of paper and roll it into a tube. This tube represents your intestines or artery. Think of the outside of the paper as your energy depot, and the inside as your intestinal/arterial lining. This lining consists of a single layer of smart cells to deal with every bite you have swallowed. It can tell "friend" from "foe," which substances to absorb and which to reject. It is also teeming with helpful bacteria, strategic partners for your gut health.

Your immune defense begins in the nose and mouth and continues in the gut. Your health works when the lining in your nose, mouth, and gut works. There are factors that can disrupt its function, as this 2014 article Intestinal Permeability—a New Target for Disease Prevention and Therapy[1] explains:

> "In particular, potential barrier disruptors such as hypoperfu-sion [reduced blood flow] of the gut, infections and toxins, but also selected over-dosed nutrients, drugs, and other life-style factors have to be considered."

Just like your skin, your gut lining can be injured. Aggravators causing acute response can include infections (e.g., *E. coli*, *Salmonella*), chronic inflammation from low oxygen (impaired mouth Structure), internal and external health disruptors mentioned earlier, and overeating. Your nose and mouth make up the admission office of them all, with you as the Director of Admissions.

What keeps your gut lining healthy? Eating healthy—wholesome foods, such as grandma's home cooking made with whole food cooked from scratch. The odds of finding health-building eats in box-stores and chain restaurants is way lower compared to shopping yourself and prepping and cooking at home. "What? You want me to cook?" I can already sense some worry.

Fast convenience and gratification over time have a health consequence: congestion and inflammation. Time spent in cooking at home is time well-spent on your gut health—see chapter 23.

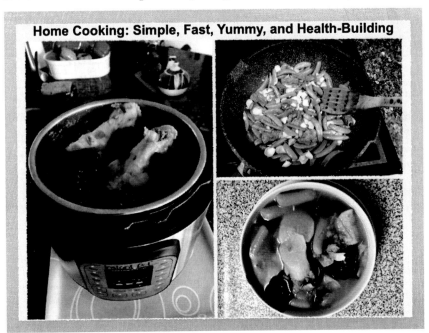

Home Cooking: Simple, Fast, Yummy, and Health-Building

Left and lower right: Soup made in a pressure cooker in 20 minutes.

Ingredients include 2 turkey wings (under $3.50), carrots, onions, mushrooms (dark), and Chinese mountain yam.

Upper right: 3-minute stir-fry with snow peas, pasture-raised beef, and chopped lotus flower root.

The Bad

"The Bad" are inflammation-inducing ingredients in packaged and prepared foods. An evidence-based 2018 Anti-inflammation Diet-101[2] lists these as gut inflamers: sugar and high fructose corn syrup, artificial trans fats, vegetable oils high in omega-6 fatty acids, refined carbs low in fiber, processed meat, and excess alcohol (2 drinks/day for men, 1 for women).

To that, I would also add antibiotics and oxygen deficiency. In the interest of brevity, we'll limit our attention to added sugars and trans-fats to represent The Bad.

A clear one-line summary is this: high fructose corn syrup (any human-added fructose) is bad for obesity and leaky gut. Simply removing added fructose can reduce diastolic blood pressure and triglyceride levels by 46% in obese children in just 10 days, reports this 2016 study[3]. Author Dr. Robert Lustig concludes, "The health detriments of sugar, and fructose specifically, are independent of its caloric value or effects on weight." He cites a telling 2012 German study[4]:

> "30% fructose solution for eight weeks [in mice] was associ-ated with the loss of the tight junction proteins occludin and ZO-1 in the duodenum [confirming increased intestinal per-meability] and a subsequent increase of bacterial endotoxin [waste from leaky gut] in the portal vein."

Translated: High fructose intake leads to leaky gut and increased bacterial toxins.

Bad fats such as artificial trans fats and canola oil are another common offender. Dr. Jerry Tennant, another highly evolved physician, offers an excellent review of the issue in *Healing Is Voltage*[5]. Here's my summary:

- Fats turn into plastic when cooked at 350° for five hours. "Fats processed in this way are called 'partially hydrogenated fats' or 'trans fats' or 'plastic fats'…When you eat these plastic fats, your cell membrane becomes made of plastic…"

- "A liver made of plastic can't clear toxins from your system. The toxins build up, causing problems such as fibromyalgia. Without a functional liver, your immune system fails, and you get all sorts of chronic infections."
- "The truth is that eating plastic fat (trans fats, canola oil) makes you fat…Your best defense is to avoid it like the plague. Go butter."

Numerous studies show that canola oil (a.k.a. rapeseed oil[6]) is toxic. One 1975 Swedish study[7] notes these effects from ingesting canola oil: growth retardation, damage to heart muscles, lowered lung capacity, lower tolerance to cold temperatures. This 1999 Brazilian study[8] showed that rats "fed the canola oils had the smallest hearts" compared to those fed a standard rat or high cholesterol diet.

The Terrible: Enablers and Perpetuators of Chronic Illness

Worse than The Bad are The Terrible: human-made chemicals that can sicken and poison your digestive organs. These include preservatives, plastics, endocrine disruptors, GMOs, pesticides, and more. Once inside your gut via the American food supply and Earth's ecosystem, they become chronic inflammation arsonists. Since wheat is a main staple in American diet, we'll focus on glyphosate, a broad-spectrum herbicide (weed killer) as representative of The Terrible.

Glyphosate now appears on the American Cancer Society's List of Probable Carcinogens[9] (Group 2A, the second strongest among 4 groups) by the International Agency for Research on Cancer. A 2019 Swedish review entitled Public Health and Evidence-Informed Policy-making: the Case of A Commonly Used Herbicide[10] notes that the addition of glyphosate to this list "resulted in high profile court cases in the USA…If a widely used herbicide turns out to be a putative cancer-causing chemical, the consequences for the producer can be potentially devastating."

As you read the rest of this chapter, ask yourself: Why and how can such a health disruptor and others be allowed to pollute our Planet Earth and your gut unchecked, until cancers set in for the courts to weight in?!

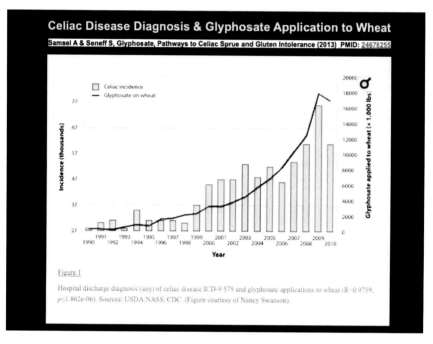

Celiac Disease Diagnosis & Glyphosate Application to Wheat

Samsel A & Seneff S, Glyphosate, Pathways to Celiac Sprue and Gluten Intolerance (2013) PMID: 24678255

Figure 1

Hospital discharge diagnosis (any) of celiac disease ICD-9 579 and glyphosate applications to wheat (R=0.9759, p≤1.862e-06). Sources: USDA/NASS; CDC. (Figure courtesy of Nancy Swanson).

Glyphosate: Gut Terrorists Embedded If Swallowed

Glyphosate was brought to use in 1974. This 2013 study[11] sheds light on glyphosate's devastating consequences:

> "Gut dysbiosis brought on by exposure to glyphosate plays a crucial role in the development of celiac disease, and more generally, gluten intolerance.
>
> Symptoms include nausea, diarrhea, skin rashes, macrocytic [oversized red blood cells] anemia and depression. It is a multifactorial disease associated with numerous nutritional deficiencies as well as reproductive issues and increased risk to thyroid disease, kidney failure and cancer."

The authors propose that glyphosate "is the most important causal factor in this epidemic—an epidemic [celiac disease and gluten intolerance] we're apt to see worsen as glyphosate residues continue to increase."

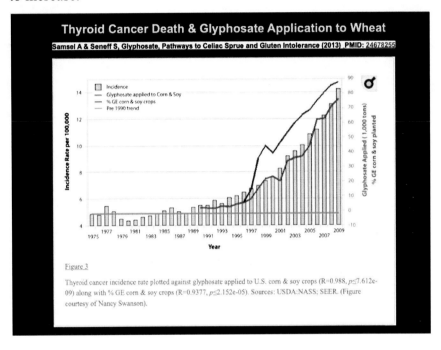

Figure 3

Thyroid cancer incidence rate plotted against glyphosate applied to U.S. corn & soy crops (R=0.988, p≤7.612e-09) along with % GE corn & soy crops (R=0.9377, p≤2.152e-05). Sources: USDA:NASS; SEER. (Figure courtesy of Nancy Swanson).

A 2016 Consensus Statement of Concern[12] likewise documented the increase in glyphosate exposure and concluded:

- Glyphosate-based herbicides (GBH) are the most heavily applied herbicide in the world and usage continues to rise;
- Worldwide, GBHs often contaminate drinking water sources, precipitation, and air, especially in agricultural regions;
- The half-life of glyphosate in water and soil is longer than previously recognized;
- GBHs are widely used on a range of crops including maize, soy grain, canola, wheat, barley, and edible beans, among others;
- Glyphosate and its metabolites are widely present in the global soybean supply;

- Human exposures to GBHs are rising; glyphosate is now authoritatively classified as a probable human carcinogen;
- Regulatory estimates of tolerable daily intakes for glyphosate in the United States and European Union are based on outdated science.

Whole wheat is more wholesome? Think again, says Dr. Stephanie Seneff[13]:

"Because the wheat is sprayed right before the harvest, it goes into the wheat germ which is the healthiest part of the wheat. It's the part that has the highest part of glyphosate contamination. Wheat bread is going to be more highly contaminated than white bread. Levels are also high on samples of legumes, chickpeas, lentils, hummus, and garbanzos from Canada and the U.S."

Quite a few patients have told me that their gluten sensitivity doesn't show up when they eat bread and pastries while on vacation in Europe. For more information, type "glyphosate use in US and Europe" or "glyphosate toxicity" into a search engine.

Tampered-with Foods: Why would I eat something that the mold won't touch?

Microbes teem over your gut cells at a 10:1 ratio. Your microbiome is your gut's strategic partner to help you digest foods, fend off infections, and make energy. This microbiome is another system of intelligence layered onto your gut on the inside, your skin on the outside, and nose and mouth in-between. Inflammation tends to show up in these sites because they make up your first line of immunity.

To reduce spoilage in large-scale American food production, pesticides and preservatives are necessary and ubiquitous. So American foods are no longer whole, nor wholesome, but tampered with.

The image below shows an organic tomato and a bun from an organic bakery that were left out (unrefrigerated) for five days. The mold on the tomato is a fungus whose task is to break down ("digest") every living thing into "ashes and dust." The mold is nature's way of recycler. Why doesn't mold touch the bun?

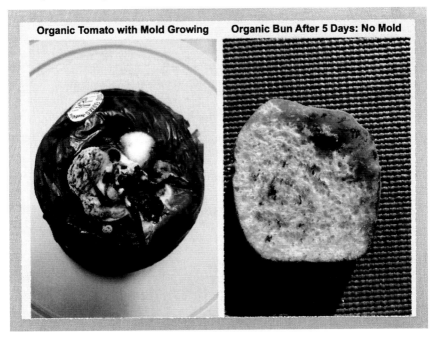

Organic Tomato with Mold Growing   **Organic Bun After 5 Days: No Mold**

Can it be that the organic bun contains something that stops the mold fungus cold? Indigestion and gut inflammation is the price of eating a tampered-with food. My money is on a fresh tomato, not a mutant bun.

WholeHealth Integration

- Your whole-body health starts with a holistic mouth Structure to support airway and sleep.

- Once you have mouth Structure, your mouth Style—how you use your mouth—spells the difference between crashing or helping your health thrive.

- Avoid foods that's been tampered with and eat only whole foods that your gut lining can accept without inflammation.

- Rule #1 in toxicology is to stop the exposure to toxins. Rule #1 in inflammation control is stop health disruptors and tampered-with foods. Since a full discussion on nutrition is beyond the scope of this primer, I recommend you seek out an expert nutritionist for guidance and coaching.

Chapter 6

Taming Your Runaway Mouth

"If I could live my life over again, I would devote it to proving that germs seek their natural habitat— diseased tissue, rather than being the cause of the diseased tissue."

~ Rudolf Virchow, MD,
Father of modern pathology

How do you celebrate a birthday, holiday, or victory? Yes, food, drink, and oral gratification is at the center of every occasion. Eating and drinking behaviors have social, environmental, and health consequences.

When stress takes a hold of you—be it a deadline, bottom line, conflict, or worry—what food/drink is your go-to? What do you reach for when fatigue gets you at work? Are the treats during a birthday or holiday celebration sweet, cold, packaged, and fast, or slow, whole, and made from scratch?

Your mouth Style can open or shut the door on opportunistic infections and degenerative diseases. It's the unhealthy internal environment that allows the germs to thrive, as Dr. Virchow suggests. The same bag of garbage left out in the open can smell very differently in mid-summer or deep winter. Some conditions breed infections, while others resist them.

You can control your internal conditions with your mouth Structure and Style. Diabetes, obesity, and/or sleep apnea can weaken the host and create "diseased tissue" which opens the window of opportunity for infections and killer diseases.

Strengthening your immune system is your best "health insurance" against illness and colds and flus. Washing hands and wearing masks are outer protections. A strong immunity provides an inner defense to fight off cancer and invaders.

You need medical expertise for snake bites or pandemics reactively. Proactively, you can empower your innate immunity with the combination of healthy mouth Structure and Style called Holistic Mouth Solutions. They provide your body with wide-open airway, quality sleep, stress mitigation, and anti-inflammation diet and bone-building nutrients.

Health Crash and Struggles Down the Road

I visited a sleep lab in the course of becoming a Diplomate in American Sleep and Breathing Academy[1] and observed three men being tested overnight. One was a lanky, retired rear admiral in his 70s, and his sleep test showed CPAP was not needed. The other two, in their 40s, both had diabetes, heart disease, a long list of medications, and potbellies that looked nine-months pregnant. They had sleep apnea (breathing stopped for 10 seconds or longer) 40 times or more per hour.

You can experience an "apnea" event yourself this way: Set your smartphone's timer for 11 seconds, then start it with your nose pinched shut and your lips zipped so no air goes in or out. It's okay to quit before the time is up if it's too challenging. How do you feel afterward? Now, imagine what 40 such events an hour can do to your heart, brain, and circulation night after night!

I also witnessed what happened when a CPAP started pushing oxygen past their obstructed airways: both men reacted with peace in their sleep. Indeed, a CPAP can be a lifesaver for such patients.

Still, the highly experienced and well-qualified technicians admit that the rejection rate of CPAP is 60-65% despite their best efforts to fit the mask to the nose.

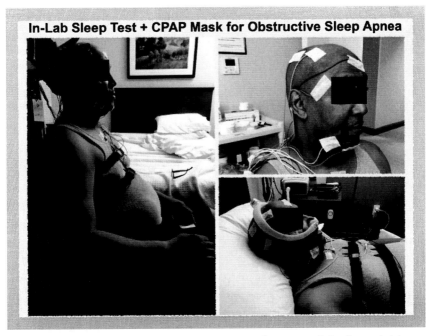

The wires and pads are for monitoring brain and body activities. The lower right image shows a Continuous Positive Airway Pressure (CPAP) mask fitted over the nose.

The gentleman pictured above was generous with his permission to share his story. His back had given out after twenty years of working as a power blaster. During that time, he ate fast and packaged foods like most construction workers and got the standard American conditions: high blood pressure, sugar, waist size. Three back surgeries later, his pain still interferes with his sleep despite an abdominal pump delivering pain medication. That is an example of a health crash.

The Source of Pot Belly and Diabetic Complications

The two potbellied men are victims of living and eating in modern America. Without training on how to eat for health, the stage is set for a cascade of health troubles: diabetes, heart disease, cancer, skin problems, allergies, toothaches, and dental infections, plus a double chin and pot belly to aggravate sleep apnea.

Diabetes and obesity come with many complications:

- "Obesity and particularly central adiposity are potent risk factors for sleep apnea," states this 2008 study[2].
- Erectile dysfunction (ED) is present in 64.4% of men diagnosed with sleep apnea, reports this 2012 study[3]. Risk factors for more severe ED include age, hypertension, and diabetes.
- Deteriorating vision and blindness can also result from diabetes, and diabetic retinopathy can raise your risk of stroke, reports new research presented at the International Stroke Conference early in 2020[4]. That risk for stroke may not be modifiable.

Taking proactive steps to prevent stroke, ED, and obesity is the only sensible strategy. Learn from the cases cited in this book and reform your mouth Style now that you know better.

Pre-Diabetes: Make Your Stand Here

"By 2012, more than a third of all US adults met the definition and criteria for metabolic syndrome," concludes a 2017 CDC report[5]. One in four American adults—and 40% of those over age 50—has at least two of the signs of pre-diabetes (a.k.a., metabolic syndrome). Here are the flashing yellow lights warning of pre-diabetes:

- Obesity
- A family history of diabetes
- High triglycerides
- High blood pressure
- High fasting blood sugar
- Low HDL (the good cholesterol)

Blindness or diabetic amputation may be down the road if you ignore them. By heeding those warnings now, you can avoid a nasty end.

Diabetes Markers and Stages

American Diabetes Association

Result	Fasting Plasma Glucose (FPG)
Normal	less than 100 mg/dl
Prediabetes	100 mg/dl to 125 mg/dl
Diabetes	126 mg/dl or higher

Result	A1C
Normal	less than 5.7%
Prediabetes	5.7% to 6.4%
Diabetes	6.5% or higher

Result	Oral Glucose Tolerance Test (OGTT)
Normal	less than 140 mg/dl
Prediabetes	140 mg/dl to 199 mg/dl
Diabetes	200 mg/dl or higher

Talk to your doctor about your blood sugar and home monitoring. Add a glucose meter to your wearable health monitors. I track my own fasting blood sugar at home to steer away from pre-diabetes. I draw my red line at the low end of pre-diabetes of 100 mg/dl. Discuss with your doctor regarding what's appropriate for you.

One day, I had a green papaya salad and crabmeat/shrimp/egg fried rice from a favorite restaurant and decided to see how my body responded. One hundred minutes after my meal, my blood sugar was 148. I limited rice in my diet after that.

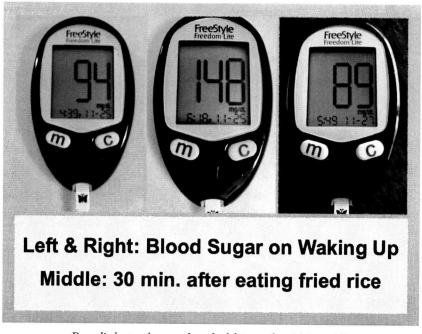

Left & Right: Blood Sugar on Waking Up

Middle: 30 min. after eating fried rice

Pre-diabetes lower threshold is under 100 mg/dl.

You can do the same for your favorite snacks or comfort foods. Test your blood sugar after snacking on your grapes, chocolates, pizza, bagel, or caramel macchiato. You may be as surprised as I was.

If you have grown up in America or lived here for many years, your taste has been conditioned for high sugar, salt, and fats, such that normal tastes bland. Processed and fast food are increasingly dominating America's food landscape and undermining consumer health. How can you stay away from America's leading killer diseases?

It's time to own up to *how* you eat. It's time to get "licensed" to head off the disasters of diabesity—the morbid combination of diabetes and obesity.

Chapter 7

A Sweet Tooth's Devastations Beyond Cavities

"Refined sugar can paralyze white blood cells for up to 5 hours."

~ Dr. David Brownstein, MD

Do you have a sweet tooth? It's a question I routinely ask my patients, because sugar goes beyond dental cavities to start many killer diseases. Indulging your sweet tooth can weaken your immunity by reducing your white blood cells' ability to "eat" microbial invaders.

This 1973 study[1] revealed: "Oral 100-g portions of carbohydrate from glucose, fructose, honey, or orange juice all significantly decreased the capacity of neutrophils to engulf bacteria…the effects last at least 5 hrs. On the other hand, a fast of 36-60 hr significantly increased the phagocytic index."

Translated: Eating sugar and its cousins can knock down your immunity for up to 5 or longer. Getting your immunity back up takes 7 to 12 times longer with fasting. Sugar gives your body a bad deal.

In the proactive spirit, let's check up on your sweet tooth with these yes/no questions:

- I have had cavities, root canals, and/or teeth pulled.
- I love anything crunchy or salty or sweet (or all three!).
- I have "love handles" or a potbelly.
- I have aches and pains that keep showing up no matter what I try.
- I feel fatigued too often. In fact, a nap right now would be great!
- I have headaches, recurring sinusitis, mouth breathing, and/or snoring.
- I have leg cramps, foot tingling, skin breakouts or itch, and/or aging spots.
- I have had a medical "-ectomy"—surgical removal of an organ, such as the gallbladder, appendix, cataract, etc.
- I have a family history of diabetes, heart disease, cancer, stroke, Alzheimer's, and/or obesity.
- I treasure my eyesight, teeth, and toes, and I'd do anything to keep them.

This survey is adapted from *Sugar Crush*[2] by Dr. Richard P. Jacoby, who offers the following score chart:

> 1 to 2 yeses: You're lying.

> 3 to 4: Not too bad, but read on.

> 5 or more: Forget the weight loss. This book [*Sugar Crush*] could save your life.

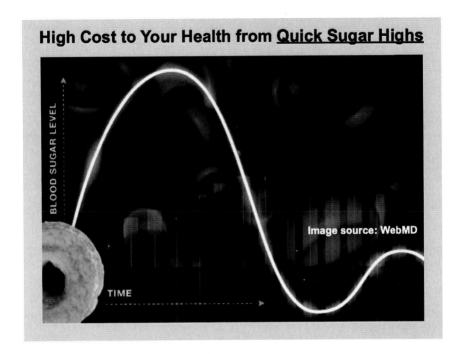

Sugar Crush

Dr. Jacoby is a podiatrist surgeon who has seen sugar's destruction up close for a career. "I am asking you to derail this express train taking you straight from sugar to peripheral neuropathy—then onward to diabetes, cardiovascular disease, stroke, and many other neurological disorders," Dr. Jacoby writes in *Sugar Crush*. With his kind permission, here are some highlights: "By the time you notice the symptoms of diabetes neuropathy from nerve compression in the tarsal tunnel of the foot, you've had uncontrolled high blood sugar for a very long time."

"Sugar crush" is the excruciating pain from diabetic neuropathy, and the culprit is eating too much sugar. "When you eat a diet heavy in processed foods full of wheat and refined sugar, your body is put on a glucose roller coaster," Dr. Jacoby explains. He continues:

> "Because the fiber has been stripped out of these products, the sugar inherent in all carbohydrates literally enters the

bloodstream in a rush. As your blood sugar spikes, most of the excess gets carried away to be stored as abdominal fat.

While that's happening, excess glucose still circulates throughout your body, attaching itself to proteins (glycating) and building up sorbitol [a byproduct of breaking down glucose] in the cells, causing them to swell and compress the nerves."

This explains leg cramps and foot pain, and "love handles," pot belly, etc. *Sugar Crush* also explains pain and dysfunction in other parts of the body where there are unyielding nerve passages: carpal tunnel, plantar fasciitis, Morton's neuroma. I believe sugar crush explains toothaches and root canals too.

Sugar/Carbs + Trauma = Pain, Neuropathy, and Possible Foot Amputation

Dr. Jacoby recalls being a young surgical student participating in his first amputation. His job was to hold a gangrenous leg that stunk up the whole room while the surgeon sawed: "But how did it get to that point?...The answer could have been so simple. Stop eating sugar."

No doctor can change your behavior. He/she is only the messenger. *You* alone have the power to stop eating excess sugar as the owner of your health.

Beware that sugar can be a tough addiction to shake once it takes hold in your brain. The following research findings may be tedious to read, but taking them to heart has been helpful for me to shed my sweet tooth. I hope you will take the time to absorb them and free yourself from sugar's powerful hook.

The Addictive Nature of Sugar

Sugar is extremely addictive and that's why it's a major additive in processed foods. "Intense Sweetness Surpasses Cocaine Rewards" is the headline of this 2007 French study[3]. Its finding: given a choice between water sweetened with saccharin and intravenous cocaine, 94% of the lab rats opted for the sweet water.

A small sampling of evidence of sugar's potent addictive potential include:

- "Sugar is noteworthy as a substance that releases opioids and dopamine and thus might be expected to have addictive potential," states Evidence for Sugar Addiction[4] in 2008. "The evidence supports the hypothesis that under certain circumstances rats can become sugar dependent. This may translate to some human conditions as suggested by the literature on eating disorders and obesity."
- "Sugar has a drug-like effect in the reward center of the brain," writes Dr. Joel Furman, MD, in The Negative Impact of Sugar on the Brain[5]. "For many people, having a little sugar stimulates a craving for more. Scientists have proposed that sweet foods—along with salty and fatty foods—can produce addiction-like effects in the human brain, driving loss of self-control, overeating, and subsequent weight gain."
- "High levels of glucose or fructose in the diet regulate the gut microbiota and increase intestinal permeability, which precedes the development of…inflammation, and lipid accumulation, ultimately leading to hepatic steatosis [fatty liver] and normal-weight obesity," as this 2018 Korean study[6] states.

Sugar excess can torpedo your health precisely because it's addictive to your brain—each mouthful re-enforces the drive to the next. Its casualties can include:

- Premature aging of the skin, says a 2012 German study[7]. Glycation is a chemical bonding of sugars (glucose or fructose) with fats or protein. Glycation makes the surface of a roast chicken crisp and golden brown, as well as brown spots and wrinkles on your face.

- Starting or worsening many degenerative diseases, such as diabetes, atherosclerosis, chronic kidney disease, and Alzheimer's, and "the increased risk of developing ED [erectile dysfunction]," found this 2013 Portuguese Review[8].
- Even in healthy young men: "Low to moderate sugar sweetened beverage consumption impairs glucose and lipid metabolism and promotes inflammation," states this Swiss trial 2011[9].
- A 3X higher risk of early death, according to a 2010 Australian study[10].
- Diabetics have a 53% greater risk of surgical site infections, reports 2016 review[11] of 94 studies.

Knowing all this research has helped me tame my own sweet tooth. For non-readers, here's a short and sweet slideshow by WebMD: "The Truth About Sugar Addiction[12]."

Americans' Lunacy for Added Sugar

The average American consumes 126 grams of sugar per day. That's a little more than three standard cans of soft drink every day and 2.5 times the recommended daily allowance.

"Americans are eating and drinking too much added sugar[13]," notes the CDC. "The leading sources of added sugars in the US diet are sugar-sweetened beverages, grain-based desserts like cakes and cookies, candy, and dairy desserts like ice cream."

Even your good-morning orange juice from a commercial carton has added sugar. "An 8-ounce (240-ml) serving of orange juice has about twice the calories and sugar of a whole orange," writes Marsha McCulloch, MS, RD, for Healthline[14]. "Their vitamin and mineral content is similar, but juice loses some vitamins and beneficial plant compounds during processing and storage."

"We all know Americans love their sugar," reported the *Washington Post* in 2015[15]. "But data from market research firm Euromonitor suggest that the love may border on lunacy, at least compared with the rest of the world." Americans consume more than double the average amount of all the other countries included in the report.

The CDC advises that added sugars make up no more than 10% of your total daily calories. At 2,000 calories a day, less than 200 of those calories should come from sugar. That's about 50 grams or 12 teaspoonfuls.

Is it okay to use honey instead of table sugar? No, honey is still sugar. One 2015 USDA Research Service[16] study showed that eating 50 grams of sugar a day for two weeks "resulted in similar effects on measures of glycemia, lipid metabolism, and inflammation," be it sucrose, honey, or high fructose corn syrup.

Monster Sugars

Sucrose is chemistry's name for table sugar, and it's 50:50 glucose and fructose. High fructose corn syrup (HFCS) is an artificial chemical made of 40:60 glucose to fructose created by the beverage industry for enhanced sweetness. Studies have shown HFCS comes with increased health risk.

"Given that Americans drink 45 gallons of soda a year, it's important for us to have a more accurate understanding of what we're actually drinking," said Michael Goran[17], PhD, of this 2014 study[18]. "We found what ends up being consumed in these beverages is neither natural sugar nor HFCS, but instead a fructose-intense concoction that could increase one's risk for diabetes, cardiovascular disease and liver disease."

Processed foods that typically contain high-fructose corn syrup include: soft drinks, candy, sweetened yogurt, frozen convenience foods and boxed dinners, bread and other baked goods, fruit juice, breakfast cereal, sauces and condiments, snack foods, cereal and nutrition bars, creamer, jams and jellies, and ice cream. How many times a day do you assault your gut and blood vessels with them? And each week, and year?

About 60% of all processed foods contain some added sugar, including foods we'd never think of as "sweets" such as packaged ketchup, chocolate milk, or spaghetti sauce. Do an online search on "unexpected foods with added sugar" and see for yourself. "The human body isn't designed to process this form of sugar at such high levels. Unlike glucose, which serves as fuel for the body, fructose is processed almost entirely in the liver where it is converted to fat," says Dr. Goran.

To stay below pre-diabetes threshold, sugar is the first item on a nutrition label that I check—not sodium (salt) or fats. If it has corn syrup (HFCS) or added sugar by any other name, it does not land in my shopping cart.

But does this mean no more sugar *ever*? That depends on whether your body is fit to handle sugar and sweets. One overweight patient complained, "You just took all the fun out of my life!"

My answer? I'm offering you a way to lower your risk of blindness, foot amputation, root-canals, etc., from cardiovascular damages of sugar overdose.

Get trained on how to wean off your sweet tooth or, as Dr. Jacoby puts it, "you can kiss your health, good looks, teeth, and body parts good-bye."

WholeHealth Integration

- Your sweet tooth can cause bitter consequences: blindness, leg amputation, brain deterioration, wrinkled face, candida and other infections, and more, from sugar overload.

- High-fructose corn syrup is toxic to children's and adults' health alike.

- Monitor your blood sugar at home. Ask your HCP if you can afford to eat added sugar in processed foods. I aim to keep my blood sugar below 95.

◆ Knowing the science behind excessive sugar's ravages can empower your cognitive brain to control ingrained impulses in your emotional brain.

Chapter 8

Hijacked and Hooked:
How Big Food's Got You

"As a kidney specialist, I know that type 2 diabetes is, by far, the biggest cause of kidney disease. After treating thousands of patients over decades, it gradually dawned on me that none of these [standard] diabetes medications actually make any real difference to the health of patients.... Whether these patients took their medications or not, they still progressed to more and more severe forms of disease. Their kidneys failed. They had heart attacks. They got strokes. They went blind. They needed amputations."

~ Dr. Jason Fung, MD,
The Diabetes Code[1]

Sugar excess is evil to health—I got it by the time I read this far into *The Diabetes Code*. Images of This is your brain on drugs[2] came to my mind: an egg (your brain) cracked open and dropped onto a sizzling pan (excess sugar).

Sugar is as addictive as cocaine to the human brain. The outcome is ugly, and the path is nasty. When your kidneys fail, you die from internal poisoning of your own cellular waste. I hope the messages from Dr. Jacoby, Dr. Fung, and myself sink in with you before it's too late. The challenge is how to wake up while you are in the jaws of addiction.

Satisfying your sweet tooth when your health can't afford to is a form of slow death just like airway obstruction in sleep apnea. While you need a doctor to help with sleep apnea, you have 100% control over how much sugar gets past your lips.

I count myself lucky, because I'd eat *all* the leftovers on the table and do it again when the next meal came in my youth. That pattern lasted until my mid-50s when I stopped doing triathlons and marathons. Still, my body paid a price for my uninformed mouth style made worse by the typical American fares—until I started writing this book.

It took me 50 years, cataract surgery in both eyes, and a few brushes with sugar crush, but I did finally get the message: rein in my own sweet tooth before diabetes and neuropathy get me. It does not mean zero sugar in my life yet, but I can stop after just a few bites with ease. That's the point of Holistic Mouth Style—knowing how to eat to enjoy life's goodies without harming yourself.

Fixing My Own Sweet Tooth

I was never a sugar-holic—endlessly nibbling chocolate, munching cookies, or chomping candy bars. But to be totally honest, I was never in full control either. How about you?

I never took sugar seriously because I was always athletic and trim, even after I became a dentist. I got through dental school starting every morning with a chocolate-iced donut and black coffee, and I did brush after each meal and floss every night. Then, I married a gifted wife who cooked from scratch, and her desserts were heavenly treats and truly irresistible.

Then came homemade hand-dipped ice cream from a local mom and pop shop with my favorite coffee flavor. Next came the imported dark chocolate bars with almond slivers. For the past twenty years, whenever I sat at my desk to write, black coffee and a piece of pastry would serve as rocket fuel for my brain.

I said "no more" after reading all those studies we looked at in the last chapter. Four days later, sugar-sober, I gloated, "In your face, Big Sugar! Ha, ha, ha! Where's your grip on me now?"

But soon after that came a baffling stumble. Fatigue got to me. So did writer's block. I was no longer so sure I could pull off this book. *This is so not like me!* Despite feeling tired after seeing patients all day, I made some soup with bone broth, Napa cabbage, homemade wonton, and freshly picked tomatoes dropped off by a patient and organic farmer—yummy (thank you Suki and Sagie)! That revived me quite a bit.

Still, when I sat down in front of my keyboard, my mind was all blank. I just could not get into my writer's realm, where ideas normally flow like a babbling brook. It was perplexing and frustrating. Suddenly, I realized that my next chapter wouldn't be ready for the publisher the next day!

Guess what I did next?

No, I didn't turn to sugar. I knew better, but I did cave into watermelon and a box of toasted seaweed. Still, I craved something else. *Am I out of my mind?!*

Changing Your Mouth Style Is an Inward Journey

"You don't need this, Felix." I recall repeating this to myself on my way to buy my favorite can of peanuts. "You don't want to do this!" It all fell on deaf ears. I was not in control, even if I was fully aware of what I was doing. Sure, the peanuts were organic and non-GMO, but I didn't stop until four ounces were gone.

So, what had happened? My emotional brain hijacked my thinking brain, and I took to eating salted peanuts over chocolates to escape my stress.

Can I afford this pattern? What would I need to do if I kept giving in time and again? "Oh, one sweet treat can't hurt me" is a self-delusion that leads to a stealthy gain around the waist and vicious consequences inside the arteries. Once I became aware, I needed to change.

Turning around your mouth style is an inward journey first, then an ongoing evolution with ups and downs until the old pattern fades. It's rarely a flip of the restart switch and clean finish. Sweet tooth is an addiction pattern that dies hard. Be kind to yourself in your expectations but be firm—keep away from guardrails and you won't go off the cliff. Keep your blood sugar low by monitoring it at home yourself with professional supervision.

Designed to Hook You: Toxic Bliss Points Built into Processed Foods

On a flight from Utah to DC, the man next to me read *The Economist* the whole way and ate all four packages of snacks offered by stewardesses, plus a king-sized bag of M&Ms. Big Food manufacturers and their marketing have won big in conditioning us consumers. Even highly educated Americans have lost that intuitive sense of what's good to eat.

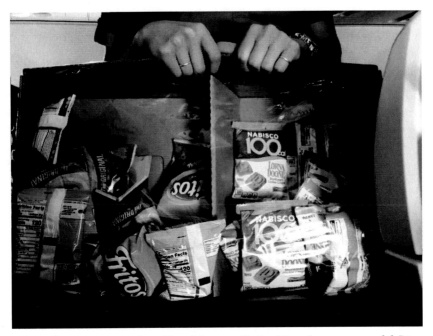

Complimentary snacks offered in one flight. Note how successful Big Food is.

"To make a new soda guaranteed to create a craving requires the high math of regression analysis and intricate charts to plot what industry insiders call the 'bliss point,' or the precise amount of sugar or fat or salt that will send consumers over the moon," writes Michael Moss in *Salt, Sugar, Fat: How The Food Giants Hooked Us*[3].

Big Food stops at nothing to get you to crave the highly tweaked "foods" inside their shiny branded package. "Don't talk to me about nutrition," said one superstar CEO quoted by Moss. "Talk to me about taste, and if this stuff tastes better, don't run around trying to sell stuff that doesn't taste good."

Sales trump nutrition. Corporate profits top customer health. You'd have to make the same choice if you were a Big Food CEO answerable to shareholders.

But consumers are the ones who pay the price after eating processed food concentrates. As Walter Willett, chair of Harvard's Department of Nutrition, explains in Moss's book, quoted here with the publisher's permission:

> "The transition of food to being an industrial product really has been a fundamental problem. First, the actual process has stripped away the nutritional value of the food. Most of the grains have been converted to starches. We have sugar in concentrated form, and many of the fats have been concentrated and then, worst of all, hydrogenated, which creates trans-fatty acids with very adverse effect on health."

Not that food company execs did not know this. Moss described a 1999 meeting of the big brass from Big Foods: "We cannot pretend food isn't part of the obesity problem," one presenter said.

> "No credible expert will attribute the rise in obesity solely to decreased physical activity. What's driving the increase [of obesity]? Ubiquity of inexpensive, good-tasting, super-sized energy-dense foods."

We've all been hooked by the toxic "bliss points" processed into the packaged foods designed to addict you. The food industry is winning in terms of bottom line, at the expense of consumers' waistlines.

"Inevitably, the manufacturers of processed food argue that they have allowed us to become the people we want to be: fast and busy, no longer slaves to the stove," writes Moss. "But in their hands, the salt, sugar, and fat they have used to propel the social transformation are not nutrients as much as weapons—weapons they deploy, certainly, to defeat their competition, but also to keep us coming back for more."

Sugar, as added in processed foods, is not a nutrient, but a hook to get you by Big Foods. It's used mercilessly to manipulate us humans with "an inborn hypersensitivity to sweet" ingredients, as a 2007 French study[4] concluded:

> "The supernormal stimulations of these receptors by sugar-rich diets such as those now widely available in modern

societies will generate a supernormal reward signal in the brain, with the potential to override self-control mechanisms and thus lead to addiction."

Beware: Sugar has been weaponized for corporate profits. The healthcare cost to you can be catastrophically severe.

WholeHealth Integration

- Sugar is as addictive as cocaine to the human brain. The fallout is nasty, and the degeneration is painful.

- Big Food manufacturers have hijacked the human brain to get us addicted to their products loaded with salt, fat, and sugar. You are in for diabetes, obesity, and health troubles if you regularly eat the standard American super-sized, energy-dense, processed or fast foods.

- Feeding your sweet tooth day after day is a form of slow death, just like sleeping with a choked airway night after night.

- Sleep apnea and choked airway require a doctor to fix, but avoiding added sugar and all its ugly cousins is 100% in your power.

Chapter 9

In Big Food's Crosshairs

"Food manufacturers, food designers, and restaurant owners may not fully understand the science behind the appeal of their foods, but they know that sugar, fat, and salt sell."

~ Dr. David A. Kessler,
The End of Overeating[1]

"Very little holds my attention the way a pizza holds my attention," said a man mentioned in Dr. Kessler's book. "I'm telling you, food talks. All food talks."

Most of us have been conditioned to behave this way by Big Food, America's processed food industry. It's been "remarkably successful at designing foods to capture the attention of people."

You are in the crosshairs of Big Food and their marketers. If you've bought their packaged products repeatedly, you've become like one of Pavlov's dogs, conditioned to salivate over the logo and motivated to pay to stay hooked.

Pavlov's Dogs: Classical Conditioning

Russian physiologist Ivan Pavlov was using dogs to study digestion in the 1890s. He noticed that the dogs would begin salivating as soon as they saw the person who usually brought them their food, not the food itself. Pavlov then designed a test. First, he'd set off a metronome. After the sound, he'd give food to the dogs. Very quickly, the dogs began to salivate as soon as they heard the metronome.

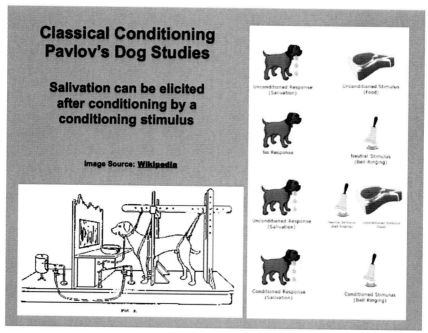

Pavlov's dogs had learned to associate the sound with food. This is called classical conditioning[2]. Interestingly, he also found that the composition of the saliva was different than that of saliva stimulated by food alone.

If your saliva starts flowing at the sight of logos or the sound of a company jingle prompts you to crave your favorite treat, that company has got you conditioned. Nutritional wisdom takes a back seat to craving created by "conditioned hyper-eating" described by Dr. David Kessler.

Conditioned Hyper-eating

"Conditioning can happen quickly," notes Dr. Kessler. With his kind permission, some key points from his revealing book are quoted here.

> "In one study, people were given a high-sugar, high-fat snack for five consecutive mornings. For days afterward, they wanted something sweet about the same time…even though they had not previously snacked at that time. Desire had already taken hold."

What can trigger your desire to eat? The smell of freshly baked bread? Meat on the grill? Coffee? The crunch of someone munching on chips? The golden crispy surface of French fries? Home-cooking reminiscent of your childhood home or country of origin?

"The cues grip us, arouse us to act," Kessler writes. "Cues ensure that we will work hard to obtain the reward. That concept is well-known in the food industry, where the most important goal of food design is to create anticipation."

When we're constantly exposed to foods engineered to trigger cravings, our brains actually change. We want more and more of the same stimulation. This can lead to what Kessler calls "conditioned hypereating."

> "How does conditioned hypereating override the executive control functions of the healthy human brain that should allow us to say no to highly palatable food? Why should a cookie be anything more than just a cookie? What explains the potency of arousal? Three powerful and interdependent forces engage fundamental neural mechanisms that interfere with executive control: cues, priming, and emotions. These

triggers amplify the beckoning power of highly palatable food and make it difficult for many people to turn away."

This is how your emotional brain is engaged. How can you counter all the sophisticated cues designed to turn on your saliva and override your "I know better"? This is why Holistic Mouth Style integrates all 3 parts of the brain in chapters 21-25.

A simple step to get unhooked from Big Food is to just turn off commercial-filled media. It's a no-cost, yet highly effective, way to calm your brain from being hyper-stimulated by their cues.

Two Potbellies Gone and One Life Nearly Lost

You don't have to remain Pavlov's dogs doomed to a lifetime of conditioned overeating on cues. You are the owner/operator of your mouth. Don't let the food companies keep you conditioned.

Turning on your common sense is another way to change your mouth Style free of charge. Even small changes in mouth Style can lead to big gains when a person takes charge of his/her mouth like a responsible driver.

One day in 1997, Reverend Myles came to my dental office for his check-up and cleaning. I could hardly recognize him—his Santa-like potbelly was gone. "Congratulations! How did you do it?" I asked.

"Oh, it wasn't that hard," he explained, beaming. "You see, five to ten times a week, I'd have events to attend as the pastor of my church: baptisms, weddings, funerals, holidays, and all. Members of my congregation were always pressing food and drinks into my hands—you know how it goes. And it had been that way for thirty years. Well, after our chat about my paunch six months ago, I simply decided to cut out the wine—and with that goes the cheese. I just asked for club soda with lemon instead."

Brilliant! Reverend Myles had used his common sense to put our chairside chat into action—no books, no Internet needed. He kept his jolly smile but changed his mouth Style, and his body responded.

Then, there was Kent. He was built tall and big. His waist was so wide, he'd have a hard time fitting his arms inside the dental chair. Yet one day he came in looking slimmer in my dental hygienist's chair.

"What happened to you? I'm impressed," I said.

"I went to a week-long Zen retreat, where we had to keep silent the whole time," Kent answered. "We were told to chew our food 60 times before swallowing. It was nearly impossible at first. I stuck with it and kept it up after I got home. The rest was easy."

Kent turned a sensible meditation exercise into a new habit. His body responded to his new mouth Style, and life with his new wife got even better.

Finally, when common sense is snuffed out by "power-through" repeatedly, big trouble can follow. Dr. Z had been a radiologist—very smart, athletic, gregarious, likable. And he loved to eat after his workouts. Then, he quit medicine to pursue a new business, and life got super busy. In 4 years' time, he accomplished enough to achieve super success so he could retire in comfort and luxury. Still, he'd always push himself to exercise after work, no matter how hard the day and how late the night.

"I don't feel so good," Dr. Z called his wife after a workout one day, and then collapsed. Luckily, his wife dialed 911 and Dr. Z survived his heart attack.

Pushing the limits takes a toll on your body, regardless of your line of work. Sacrificing your health in pursuit of wealth has too many sad endings. Real success is the quality of your journey.

If you've made it financially, be sure to keep what you've got. Stay well.

WholeHealth Integration

- Big Foods commercials have successfully hyper-conditioned us consumers to salivate like Pavlov's dogs to eat their overloaded foods designed to hook you.

- Turning off your TV/smartphone and turning on your common sense can help you adopt holistic mouth Style with greater ease and effectiveness.

- You don't need an advanced degree to turn from unknowingly harming your health to a caring and successful owner-operator of your mouth, as Rev. Myles and Kent did.

- Stop killing yourself like Dr. Z did once you've secured your financial future—see Resources for Smart Health Keeping™ webinars and workshops.

- Smart retirement/financial planning should include (1) ensuring your mouth structure can support alignment, breathing, circulation, and sleep, and (2) getting "licensed" to eat well and eat right to reduce obesity and inflammation early on.

Chapter 10

Your Mouth Style Checkup and Inside-Out Change

"I've been surprised to find that unraveling the determinants of overeating has required me to consider psychology, philosophy, economics, neuroendocrinology, history, labor, and government regulation."

~ Kima Cargill, PhD,
The Psychology of Overeating[1]

Overeating is too easy, but controlling it can be complicated, as Dr. Cargill discovered. Stuffing food down is a no-brainer, but eating to thrive takes all three parts of our human brain.

So, let's start with this foundational question: *Why* do you eat? This determines whether your health thrives or crashes. Do you eat to support your health with pleasure or to support your pleasure at the cost of your health? Do you eat to nourish or trash your body?

Mouth Style as used here is how you choose to keep your health and operate your mouth. When your rational mind is in control, you behave logically. But what happens when your emotional stress takes over?

What's Driving Your Mouth to Act Out?

When you're stressed, what do you do to make yourself feel better? Do you eat? Drink alcohol? Do you argue, cry, or yell? Talk with a friend? Exercise? Chew on your nails or bite your lips or tongue? Sleep? Smoke? Talk with a therapist? Swallow your feelings?

Those are the answers from 11,000 people who were surveyed by *Prevention Magazine* in 1995[2]. Nearly all these stress reactions involve the mouth in some way, including the swallowing of feelings.

The mouth is where stress shows up. Keep that point in mind the next time you're tempted to reach for that dark chocolate, soda, or pretzel.

Eating: 'The Dominant Stress Response'

Stress predictably induces a drive to use the mouth. Stress eating, drinking, smoking, and binging are forms of self-comfort leading to inflammation and obesity.

This oral response to stress was documented in a 1975 study[3] in which rats were subjected to mild stress via having their tails pinched by a hemostat locked at the first notch one inch from their tails' ends. "The tail pinch," the researchers wrote, "preferentially elicited the oral responses of eating, gnawing, and licking in intact, [food]-sated rats."

The most common response was eating, even though the rats had already been fed: "Such oral responses were universal" and "were initiated a few seconds after tail-pinch began." They tended to last until the pinch was over, sometimes longer.

A 2014 *The Burden of Stress in America*[4] survey found that roughly half of all Americans reported "a major stressful event or experience in the past year." Of those people, 43% reported "stressful events and experiences related to health."

So, what's pinching your tail? This is a useful check the next time you feel driven to eat, drink, argue, snap, cry, shut your mouth, or swallow your feelings.

Stress Eating Illustrated

Once, I had been teaching and traveling for four days straight before flying back in a redeye to see patients on Monday morning. I powered through the morning, but tiredness crept in with three patients to go. That led me to do something very atypical: I had a cheap cup of coffee from a fast-food chain, plus two mini pies!

"Don't do this, Felix!" I said to myself in the elevator down. "Think it through and turn back." That warning from my rational brain did not stop me. I got the coffee and wolfed down both pies like a freshman newly home from college. Within minutes, I could feel my heart rate going up—a sign of stress in my already tired body.

What had happened? I didn't eat the pies because of hunger. I had just filled my belly with steak over rice with a yummy sauce for lunch. But confronted with stress—having more work than energy— my emotional brain had kidnapped my judgment. My tail had been pinched, and I responded with irrational eating—again! My mouth style was still a work in progress.

Of course, an occasional stray is okay, though it still comes at a bodily cost. And those costs can skyrocket into real health troubles when exceptions become routines, such as having a Thanksgiving feast every Sunday.

Taking Stock of Your Body and the Habits Feeding It

Body mass index (BMI) is used by doctors to classify a person's weight as underweight, normal, overweight, or obese. If you don't already know your BMI, click here[5].

Although those labels may sound judgmental, BMI doesn't come with shame or criticism. It's just a number indicating the status of your weight in relation to your height. Be aware that your BMI may change with age. As the CDC tells it, "The proportion of muscle decreases and fat increases. This shift slows their metabolism, making it easier to gain weight."

Bottom line: "Raised BMI also increases the risks of cancer of the breast, colon, prostate, endometrium, kidney and gallbladder," says WHO[6].

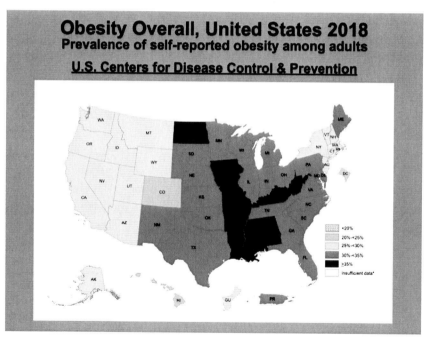

Now, let's get more specific by looking into your typical week of 20 meals (with a Sunday brunch for round numbers). How many times a week do you:

- Eat fast food or convenience/packaged/take-out foods?
- Eat breakfast in a rush or not eat at all?
- Eat lunch on the go, with your eyes glued to a screen or while multitasking?
- Feel sleepy after lunch?
- Overeat at dinner?
- Eat dinner 4 hours or more before sleep?
- Get less than 7 hours of sleep?
- Wake up in the morning feeling tired?

Now, compare your answers to the following research conclusions:

- "Over 36% (1 in 3) Americans eat fast food on a given day," reports USA Today reported in 2018[7].
- "For adults, the research is undeniably clear in terms of the link between fast food consumption and weight gain," reports University Health News[8].
- Sleep deprivation is linked to weight gain and diabetes risk in this 2007 study Metabolic Consequences of Sleep Deprivation[9] via 3 pathways: 1) alterations in glucose metabolism (less effective sugar clearance), 2) overeating, and, 3) decreased energy expenditure (too little exercise).
- Sleep deprivation affects weight gain through two hormones controlling appetite: leptin (for satiety) and ghrelin (for hunger). Leptin levels go up during sleep. Insufficient sleep means lower leptin levels, triggering feelings of hunger and a general slow-down of your metabolism, explains Julia Layton in Is Lack of Sleep Making Me Fat?[10]

Now I understand why my eating went crazy the day after I flew the red-eye back to work. Sleep deprivation leads to overeating, higher stress hormones, and more insulin resistance—a precursor to diabetes—which combine to promote weight gain despite your diet and exercise.

Dinner Time, Sleep Time, and the Chinese Body Clock

There are twenty-four hours a day and twelve acupuncture meridians in the human body. From these, Traditional Chinese Medicine (TCM) evolved a body clock to connect your internal organ systems with the circadian rhythm, or the day-night cycle.

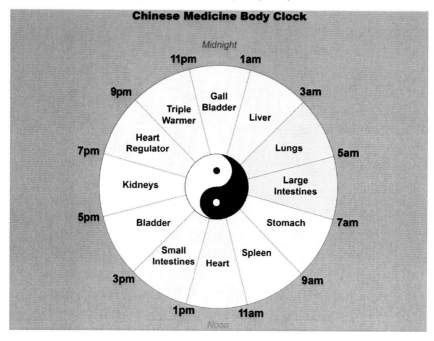

The hours of 11 p.m. to 7 a.m. are when the body does its housekeeping, while Stomach meridian (breakfast) starts the day from 7 a.m. to 9 a.m. What happens during those late night and early morning hours?

11 p.m. to 1 a.m. is Gallbladder time. This meridian aids in digestion of fats and provides lubrication to the intestines. It's associated with the emotion of frustration.

- 1 a.m. to 3 a.m. is Liver time. The liver is the most important detox organ in the body and is in charge of the emotion of anger.

- 3 a.m. to 5 a.m. is Lung time. Your lungs are in charge of breathing and involved with sleep apnea and the emotion of grief.
- 5 a.m. to 7 a.m. is Colon time. This meridian is in charge of the removal of bodily waste, as well as the emotion of being judgmental and the anal-retentive personality.
- 5 p.m. to 11 p.m. is a restorative time for Kidney, Heart Regulator, and Triple Warmer (immune system) meridians to power those vital organs and functions. From the TCM perspective, 5 p.m. to 11 p.m. is not an ideal time to exercise or work hard to burn energy. It's the time to stand down to recharge your battery.

Western science now has evidence to support the Chinese body clock concept. "Food intake is coordinated to cellular metabolism by clock gene expression with a master clock in the suprachiasmatic nucleus synchronized by light exposure," says a 2013 Australian study[11]. "Thus, gastric vagal mechanoreceptors [in the stomach] display circadian rhythm, which may act to control food intake differentially at different times of the day."

Functional Medicine: One Piece in WholeHealth Puzzle

There's another consequence of our modern lifestyle of staying indoors year-round with artificial lights and losing touch with the four seasons. Do discuss your vitamin D levels and vitamin B supplementation with your doctor or HCP.

"Vitamin D goes low (< 30 ng/ml), sleep goes bad, illness begins, repair stops, aging starts.," explains neurologist Dr. Stasha Gominak, MD, founder of RightSleep[12]. "We propose the hypothesis that sleep disorders have become epidemic because of widespread vitamin D deficiency," Dr. Gominak reports in her 2012 study[13]. "Most patients had improvement in neurologic symptoms and sleep but only through maintaining a narrow range of vitamin D3 blood levels of 60-80 ng/ml."

In her 2016 study[14], Dr. Gominak reported, "Three things did not improve with D support: irritable bowel, pain, and weight... Three months of vitamin D plus B100 (100mg of all B vitamins except 100mcg of B12 and biotin and 400mcg of folate) resulted in improved sleep, reduced pain and unexpected resolution of bowel symptoms."

With that piece of the puzzle in place, let's check out some road hazards in the form of health disruptors that commonly enter through the mouth.

WholeHealth Integration

+ Eating is the dominant stress response. Know what's pinching your tail first.

+ The day-night circadian rhythm that's hardwired into the human brain. Go to sleep by the Chinese Body Clock to get paid back with thriving health.

+ Traditional Chinese medicine excels in diagnosing and restoring Yin-Yang imbalance. Seeing an acupuncturist can help you build health and maintain wellness in ways Western science cannot, particularly when seasons change.

+ Your functional medicine doctor can support your sleep quality and chronic pain with testing and supplementation of vitamins D, B, and possibly more.

+ Big Foods have ultra-sophisticated ways to hook you and keep you addicted to the packaged foods they have tampered with.

+ Indulging your sweet tooth can torpedo your circulatory system and sink your health. Take weaning yourself off added sugar seriously.

Chapter 11

How Your Health Abandons You

When I asked Fermin [the gardener] why he cared so much about the roots, he simply smiled, "Boy," he said, "that's the way nature designed it. Your tree's health and disease start in its roots." ... After eight years of medical school, six years of training, and another fifteen years of practice, I am to the conclusion that good medicine is very much like good gardening.... If you want to get your tree truly healthy, you can't just cover up the problem. You need to get to the root of it.

~ Alejandro Junger, MD,
Clean Gut[1]

Your mouth is the port of entry into your gut and a major source of illness or wellness. Thriving or fading health literally hinges on how you operate your jaw joints. Your mouth Style is not only what you eat, how often, how fast, and how much, but also what toxins and chemicals you allow past your lips unknowingly.

In this chapter, we will look at how ingesting some foods grown in modern America can build gradually toward a health catastrophe. That's because our farms are increasingly sprayed with chemicals and our foods are altered. Just try to pronounce the ingredient list on an ice cream carton!

Gut inflammation and subsequent degeneration is inevitable from eating such foods that have been processed and altered—no longer whole. With each mouthful, you may be ingesting toxins, and parts of you may be exquisitely sensitive to them without your knowing, such as your thyroid gland to plastics and your brain to lead and mercury.

You can still enjoy eating if you know what to look for, where to shop, and when to say "no" and "no more"—that's the point of this chapter.

Meta-Inflammation and Obesity at Its Source

Meta- is a Greek prefix meaning after or beyond. Meta-inflammation is "defined as low-grade, chronic inflammation orchestrated by metabolic cells in response to excess nutrients and energy" in this 2011 Harvard article in The Annual Review of Immunology.[2] "The discovery that obesity itself results in an inflammatory state in metabolic tissues ushered in a research field that examines the inflammatory mechanisms in obesity."

Again, obesity means inflammation, which starts a series of health troubles. These will continue until the roots of obesity are addressed—your mouth Style.

"I'm tired of spending my hard-earned money on my daughter's leukemia and now my own kidney disease, taking poison pills, unable to enjoy my golden years." That from a family member after living in America for more than 50 years. Not knowing how to eat in this land of abundance got him into these troubles.

He was an impressive eater in his youth, and we were both ice cream monsters as new arrivals in America. Unlike myself, he was not athletic and mid-life brought him a pot belly, followed by diabetes, cataract surgery, a small stroke that left him unable to tuck his shirt inside his pants, and medications. All these conditions have worn out his kidneys and put hardship on his wife.

Your body has its own accounting system that amounts to a biography of your biology. How you eat leaves an internal trail just like rings in tree trunks. A happier ending of your biography starts with a review of your mouth Style.

Can You Use Holistic Mouth Style Training?

When an arrow misses the target, the archer can blame the wind or the target. Or, he/she can look inward and ask: *What can I change to better hit the bullseye next time?* In that spirit, take a minute to survey your habitual mouth Style by noting how many of the following statements apply to you:

- I reach for comfort food and/or drink when I feel stressed.
- I often multitask while I eat (watch TV, drive, play with smartphone, etc.).
- I have a sweet tooth.
- I give in to my food cravings (salt, sweet, crunchy, bubbly, etc.) every day.
- I usually/always drink cold or iced drinks with my meals.
- I frequently overeat and don't feel good afterward.
- I eat out or get take-out/delivery 5 times a week or more.
- My clothing size has been creeping up over the past 3 years.
- I value natural health above drugs and surgery.
- I love to eat, and I'd love to know how to eat without trashing my health.

The closer you come to 10, the more you need to get licensed to thrive, but any single one of them is reason enough. And the earlier you start, the better your shot at fully enjoying life.

Chapter 12

Toxins Poisoning Earth Mother and Our Children

"Will you teach your children what we have taught our children? That the earth is our mother? What befalls the earth befalls all the sons of the earth. This we know: the earth does not belong to man, man belongs to the earth. All things are connected like the blood that unites us all."

~ Chief Seattle[1], 1854

Be true to your teeth or they will be false to you. People with missing or false teeth know this all too well. Similarly, honor your mouth-gut-brain axis on the inside and our gardens and farms on the outside, or risk harming your health and your children's.

Your mouth is the admission office between your internal and outer environments. All humans, regardless of ethnic and geographic origin, are children of Mother Earth. Healthy children can only

143

come from healthy mothers. Now, Nature has been contaminated by manmade toxins which are coming back to haunt us as health disruptors. Higher levels of pollutants such as DDT, PCBs, and flame retardants (found in your sofas, car seats, and mattresses) are associated with impaired fetal growth and adult wellness.

What Have We Done to Our Children?

The offspring of women with the highest levels of a dioxin-like PCB mixture had a fetal head circumference 6.6 mm (about 1/4 inch) smaller than those with the lowest levels, reports a 2019 study[2]. The same holds with organochlorine pesticides: "a 4.7 mm reduction in fetal head circumference, a 3.5 mm reduction in abdominal circumference…"

Do you find it acceptable that your children and grandchildren grow below their potential? "These chemicals take a long time to degrade," said coauthor Pauline Mendola. "Even though most are banned, some for decades, we still see effects. Typically, people are exposed through diet and also drinking water."

Speaking of drinking water, know this if you or your favorite take-out place cooks with tap water: "pharmaceuticals pass through water treatment," U.S. Geological Survey says in 2018[3]. "Many of the more than 4,000 prescription medications used for human and animal health ultimately find their way into the environment."

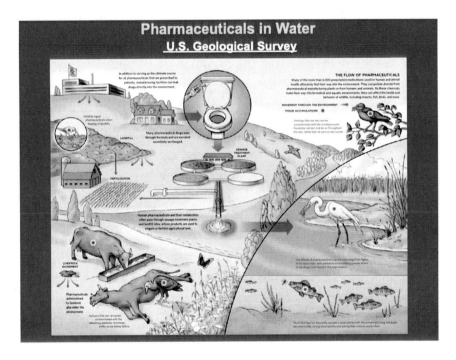

The evidence of the biological harm done to the "web of life" by human-made pollutants is shockingly widespread and ignored. Here are a few examples:

> **Plastics Filled Oceans**[4]: As a May 2019 feature in National Geographic[5] put it, the microplastics now strewn throughout our oceans is a threat "not just to young marine life, but to a broader ecosystem that relies on healthy stocks of young fish.… Plastic waste is impacting our oceans and our land on a massive scale."
>
> **Endocrine Disruptors in Pregnant Women:** "Research shows that virtually every pregnant woman in the U.S. has at least 43 different environmental chemicals in her body," reports the Plastics Pollutions Coalition[6]. "Of particular concern is exposure to known endocrine disrupting chemicals, which are found in food packaging, pesticides, cosmetics and household products, including chemical coatings."

Babies Are Born Pre-Polluted "to a disturbing extent," as "numerous environmental contaminants can cross the placental barrier," says the 2008-09 *President's Cancer Panel Report*[7]. "Opportunities for eliminating or minimizing cancer-causing and cancer-promoting environmental exposures must be acted upon to protect all Americans," it goes on to state, "but especially children."

The International Federation of Gynecology and Obstetrics[8] has noted: "Exposure to toxic environmental chemicals during pregnancy and breastfeeding is ubiquitous and is a threat to healthy human reproduction. There are tens of thousands of chemicals in global commerce, and even small exposures to toxic chemicals during pregnancy can trigger adverse health consequences. Documented links between prenatal exposure to environmental chemicals and adverse health outcomes span the life course and include impacts on fertility and pregnancy, neurodevelopment, and cancer."

Be true to our Planet Earth or risk mutations and extinction. Today's children are incubating in toxic wombs. It's time to wake up and help our Earth Mother recover. "Change can happen when small acts, taken together, bring powerful results," as Jean Case of National Geographic[9] says.

Leadership Lacking

California's wildfires get bigger, and Atlantic hurricanes get stronger by the year, and 100-year storms are more and more common. More than one billion animals are estimated dead from 2019 Australia fires. What have we done to Planet Earth and all life forms on it?

"Man did not weave the web of life," Chief Seattle admonished. "He is merely a strand in it. Whatever he does to the web, he does to himself." As a new grandpa in 2020, I care deeply about the increasingly sick Mother Earth we are handing over to our offspring.

What feeds your gut comes from our Mother Earth, and She's running a fever. Germs grow faster at higher temperature. It doesn't take a

PhD microbiologist to know that. One definition of incubation[10] is "the process or period of time in which harmful bacteria or viruses increase in size or number in a person's or animal's body but do not yet produce the effects of disease." The key elements of infections are all temperature dependent: the microbes, their multiplication, the host, and the lead time before symptoms.

No responsible leader should be surprised by increased infectious diseases from global warming. Denying simply aggravates wildfires and accelerates infections. The job of leaders is to lead—to get in front of issues (not just TV cameras), to foresee problems coming, and to put plans in place and solutions in motion proactively.

Poor outcome reflects poor leadership. The true measure of a real leader is not rhetoric, but extraordinary outcome in controlling environmental toxins, global warming, and pandemics. The health of our children and Planet is at stake.

Health Disruptors: Glyphosate, Plastics, Estrogen

Health disruptors are toxins or conditions that interfere with your body's ability to run its own house, or self-regulate. Your endocrine system is a major player in your body's self-regulation, and it's highly sensitive to health disruptors.

Health disruptors can include physical issues such as a choked airway, sweet tooth, hypothyroidism, mental issues like chronic stress, and chemical toxins such as pesticides, plasticizers, herbicides, and more.

Glyphosate, one of the most widely used herbicides, was detected in every wheat-based food tested by the Environmental Work Group in this 2019 study[11]. Its impact on the environment and human health is just coming to light 4 decades later. In their 2017 study[12] published in the *Journal of Biological Physics and Chemistry*, Drs. Samsel and Seneff point to one possibility:

"Glyphosate, acting as a non-coding amino acid analogue of glycine, could erroneously be integrated with or incorporated into protein synthesis in place of glycine, producing a defective product that resists proteolysis [protein digestion]. Whether produced by a microbe or present in a food source, such a peptide could lead to autoimmune disease through molecular mimicry."

That explains the increased gluten intolerance in patients. The U.S. Government allows 5.8 times more glyphosate in American foods compared to the European Union.

If you want thriving health, then beware of a whole bunch of health disruptors in modern American foods: industrial pollutants, pesticides, food preservatives, GMOs (genetically modified organisms), burgers and steak from industrial meats[13] raised in "unmatched squalor," chicken[14] raised with antibiotics and hormones, and toxic wheat[15] contaminated with glyphosate (RoundUp) that's also in breakfast foods aimed at children[16].

Consider the ubiquitous plastics commonly used to package food and beverages. Just look inside the trash you take out. As Dr. Jerry Tennant explains in *Healing Is Voltage*[17]:

"In the human body, plastic acts like estrogen…Estrogen unopposed by progesterone blocks zinc, magnesium, and vitamin B6 and leads to increases in heart attacks and strokes, aging, anxiety, allergies, asthma, breast cancer, cervical cancer, cold hands and feet, decreased sex drive, dry eyes, endometriosis, fat gain around the hips, fatigue, fibrocystic breasts, foggy thinking, gallbladder disease, hair loss, headaches, hypoglycemia, increased blood clotting, autoimmune disorders."

Ladies: How many of the above symptoms do you have? Healthcare professionals: How many of your patients do not have said signs and symptoms?

Gentlemen: You are not immune, either. "All males and females in developed nations have estrogen dominance," writes Dr. Tennant. He continues:

> "Estrogen dominance can be caused by soy, petrochemicals, fuel exhaust we breathe, propylene glycol (deodorants), sodium lauryl sulfate in toothpaste and ointments, herbicides, and pesticides. These potent estrogenic substances block the production of thyroid hormone and greatly magnify the incidence of estrogen-dependent cancers."

Estrogen dominance blocks thyroid hormone production, which explains why hypothyroidism runs rampant—see next chapter. Polluting our environment translates into poisoning ourselves.

One simple way to start reducing plastics is to substitute disposables with reusables (e.g., a thermos, refillable water bottles) or recyclable substitutes (e.g., paper straws). You can vote with your pocketbook and avoid fast/convenience food packaging to save our Earth Mother from further man-made poisons.

"What can I do for you today?" the barista asked me. "A small cup of black coffee, please," I said (pre-COVID). "Just put it straight in my thermos. I'd like to save a paper cup and avoid tasting the plastics in the cup lining."

She smiled. "I totally appreciate your concern. What a great idea!"

Regular folks get it. Now, make sure your government does its job to protect your children by cleaning up our Planet Earth.

WholeHealth Integration

- Our outer environment affects personal health more than we know, and COVID-19 reveals that all people on this planet are more connected than we can imagine.

- Your mouth is the major port of entry of environmental toxins to disrupt your reproductive and hormonal systems. What is your admission policy of what gets in? How much is okay with you and your kids?

- Be true to your environment, or thriving health will abandon you and your children.

- Vote to protect our natural environment and children, and choose where you shop and what you buy: *"What befalls the earth befalls all the sons of the earth. This we know: the earth does not belong to man, man belongs to the earth."*

Chapter 13

Hypothyroidism:
Tired, Cold, and Puffy

"A 1°C drop in our body temperature [1.8° F] will cause our immune function to decline by 40% and a low body temperature will create an environment where various diseases can be active in our body."

~ Nobuhiro Yoshimizu, MD, PhD,
The Fourth Treatment for Medical Refugees[1]

Death is a cold body, while fever is an immune response to kill viruses. Life with health exists in a narrow zone of body temperature regulated by your thyroid gland. No matter how hot or cold it is outside, your body regulates its temperature around 98°F (37°C) for optimal function. "Without thermoregulation, the human body would not be able to adequately function and, inevitably, will expire," states Physiology, Temperature Regulation[2].

151

Do you have cold hands and feet, creeping weight gain, hair falling out in clumps, the outer-third of your eyebrow missing, frequent infections, and chronic fatigue? If yes, your thyroid and adrenals may need help. Higher temperature means higher energy and greater immune power against diseases and infections.

With one look and a handshake (before COVID-19), I can pretty much tell if a new patient is prone to sleep apnea, obesity, and a bumpier road ahead. About 4.6% of the U.S. Population ages 12 and older have hypothyroidism, per NIH[3]. In my practice, I make referrals every day for thyroid and adrenal evaluation and treatment to better support oral appliance therapy for Impaired Mouth Syndrome.

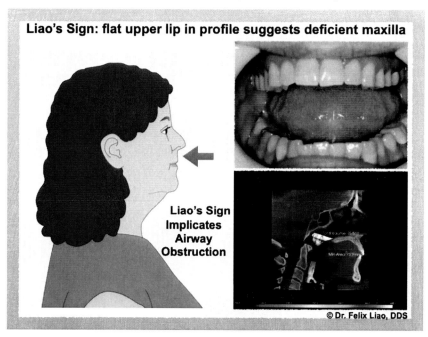

Liao's Sign: flat upper lip in profile suggests deficient maxilla

Liao's Sign Implicates Airway Obstruction

© Dr. Felix Liao, DDS

Swollen hypothyroid tongue and off-the-scale narrow airway (in black zone beyond red) in a patient with Liao's Sign implicating failure to thrive in the upper jaw.

Why is a mouth doctor harping on about your thyroid? For starters, low thyroid means lower energy and lower tolerance to the tiny 1/4 millimeter stretch from epigenetic oral appliance. Also, hypothyroid patients are more susceptible to being overweight, which aggravates sleep apnea with a super-sized "tiger" tongue.

Further, it's wise to rule out hypothyroidism first because it has overlapping symptoms with sleep apnea. Sixty-four percent of patients (124 out of 200 total) tested in a sleep center had obstructive sleep apnea, and three of the OSA patients had undiagnosed hypothyroidism in this 1999 Canadian study[4]. Both the OSA and hypothyroidism "resolved simultaneously" when their hypothyroidism was treated with thyroxine.

Your thyroid gland is located just below your Adam's apple, where it serves as your body's thermostat and the spark plug for your metabolism. Your weight, muscle strength, and even your mood are all affected by your thyroid.

Frequent symptoms of a hypothyroidism[5] (low) include weight gain, insomnia, dry skin, poor memory, bouts of anger, hair loss, sugar and caffeine craving, cold intolerance, and constipation. Why constipation? The gallbladder makes bile which serves as a lubricant to facilitate bowel movement. What if your gallbladder cells don't have enough energy? Just poor digestion, bloating, creaky and achy joints, and constipation.

Every cell in the body has receptors for thyroid hormone to make energy. That includes growing a wider maxilla and renewing your body from daily wear and tear. "Thyroid hormones both stimulate the cellular energy production necessary for life, as well as maintain our bodies' relative constant temperature," writes Mark Starr, MD in *Type 2 Hypothyroidism*[6], which has a chapter called "Environmental Toxins = Hormones Havoc" that I highly recommend.

Body Temperature and Immunity

Your body temperature matters greatly in your resistance to infections. "If our body temperature is around 36°C (96.8°F), our body will have a sufficient amount of immune functions. However, if our body temperature is around 35°C (95°F), our immune functions will decline," writes Dr. Yoshimizu, Director of Japan's Nakamachi Garden Clinic, in *The Fourth Treatment for Medical Refugees* (p. 61).

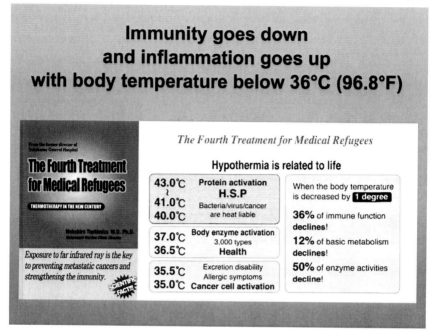

There's a whole proactive wellness strategy in this table, which is re-produced with permission of RichWay International.

A 1°C drop in temperature results in 50% decline in enzyme activity, as shown in the slide above. Since enzymes help speed biochemistry reactions to completion, lower body temperature means indigestion, food sensitivities, leaky gut, and chronic inflammation.

Living with a lower body temperature by 1°C/2°F amounts to driving a car with a sputtering engine blowing black smoke. Hypothyroidism means a body less able to respond to challenges of mouth Structure and Style change with ease.

Optimal temperature fans "stomach fire," a barometer of vitality in Traditional Chinese Medicine. It is frequently doused by peculiar American eating style.

Iced Water Aggravates Symptoms

Debilitating pain caused one of my patients to call me one Friday night. Nancy said, "I couldn't do anything this morning, not even to get into my car to see my chiropractor. Even after my sister drove me there, chiropractic didn't help."

Up until that point, Nancy had done amazingly well with her back pain using her oral appliance. I sent her to my WholeHealth acupuncturist who had treated Nancy for her back pain from several car accidents. This time, the acupuncturist found:

- Nancy had eaten dairy and cheese against the acupuncturist's advice.
- Nancy hadn't been doing the suggested posture and breathing exercises.
- Nancy had low stomach acid and drank lots of ice water with every meal.

Dairy is congestive, and ice-cold is contractive. That is another recipe for pain, on top of her hypothyroidism that was not being adequately controlled, as evidenced by her growing obesity.

Nancy's back pain went away at the end of her acupuncture visit. But what had brought it on? It was her habitual mouth Style, and Nancy learned this lesson the hard way: "Ice water is an old habit, but I did not take it seriously as a pain threat. I love cheese, and I just cheated. Now, I know the consequences."

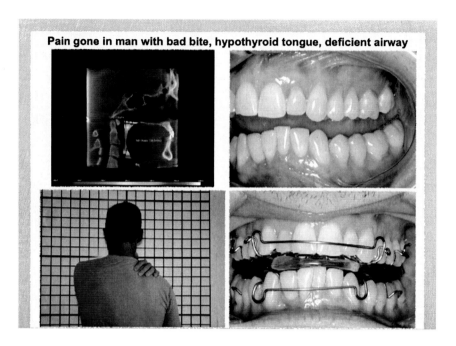

Pain gone in man with bad bite, hypothyroid tongue, deficient airway

A patient's husband had a throbbing toothache while I was teaching out of state. So, my patient sent him straight to our all-purpose acupuncturist, who in turn noted that he drank ice water all the time—including with meals. His toothache went away with acupuncture around his navel; nothing near his mouth.

Surprise—some toothache (in the absence of cavity or abscess) can originate outside the mouth and thus can be fixed without a drill or a pill—see chapter 11 on Dental Angina in *Early Sirens*. But again, why did pain start?

Think about how your neck, shoulder, and back muscles tense up—even shiver—when you go out on an icy winter day. Contraction is how your body reacts to ice-cold drinks in your core. Chronic muscle cramps from repeated shivering can result in trigger points referring pain from body to teeth.

Hypothyroid Supersizes Your Tongue

As mentioned, the tongue as a "6-foot tiger" inside a "3-foot cage" provided by under-sized jaws contributes to airway obstruction. Deficient jaw development forces the tongue into the throat, choking the airway and cutting off oxygen.

With hypothyroidism's tendency for weight gain, that "tiger" is super-sized to an 8-foot tongue inside a 3-foot mouth to initiate or aggravate sleep apnea.

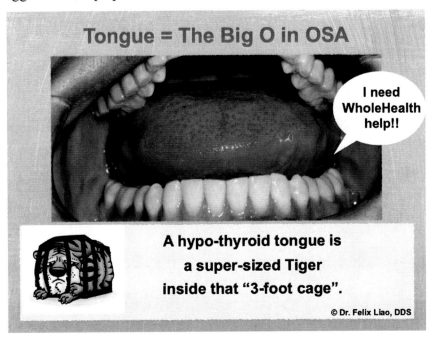

The hypothyroid tongue swells because of excessive mucin, a goo-like substance that accumulates in the tissues, resulting in a doughy facial appearance and body shape. Fifty times the normal amount of mucin was found in the skin of one woman who had died of hypothyroidism, wrote Dr. Starr.

"Mucin is like clear Karo syrup," writes Dr. Tennant in *Healing as Voltage*[7]. When you make mucin, it begins to fill your whole body with "goo" in a characteristic pattern:

- The face becomes round.
- There's a pouch under the chin.
- The shoulders appear that you're wearing shoulder pads.
- The chest becomes shaped like a barrel.
- Breasts become pendulous.
- You become bigger around the waist than the hips ("beer belly").
- The buttocks become large and wide.
- The thighs touch in the middle of the legs.

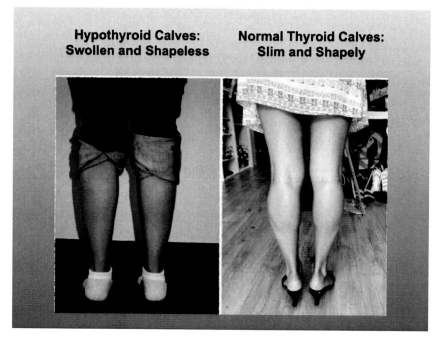

Mucin from hypothyroid is the difference between the calves of these two ladies. The one on the right grew up in Asia and continues to eat a diet rich in iodine in Hawaii.

Hypothyroidism Undermines Your Mouth Style Makeover

With hypothyroidism comes fatigue that defies nutritional or sleep apnea therapy because the energy-producer called mitochondria inside each cell is also impaired. "No matter what you eat or how much you exercise," writes Dr. Starr, "your health will suffer without proper thyroid function."

With that fatigue comes sugar craving and overeating to compensate, further exacerbating the overweight that plagues hypothyroid patients. With impaired mouth style comes poor gut health from environmental toxins, partially digested foods, and drugs (antibiotics and steroids). Worse yet, a supersized hypothyroid tongue leads to oxygen deficiency favoring the growth of bad bacteria. Now, you have a vicious cycle: Bad gut perpetuates poor thyroid.

"A whopping 20 percent of thyroid function depends on a sufficient supply of healthy gut bacteria to convert T4 to T3 [the active thyroid hormone]," says Dr. Kharrazian in Good Thyroid Health Depends on Good Gut Health[8].

Most Americans have Type 2 hypothyroidism "Because [of] fluoride in their toothpaste, visits to the dentist, etc.," writes Dr. Tennant in *Healing Is Voltage.*

The most common source of fluoride is tap water from your municipal supply. That's the risk of eating out often. For more information, search for fluoride on Mercola.com[9] or visit Fluoride Action Network[10].

Dysfunctional Liver and Chronic Illness Recovery

Your liver is a key player in your immune system. "A high cholesterol level means your body is trying to clean itself, or you have low hormones," explains Dr. Tennant in *Healing Is Voltage.* "Most of the hormones are made from cholesterol. When the liver notices that you are hormone deficient it makes more cholesterol to help you make more hormone…A chronically ill patient has a dysfunctional liver clogged with trans fats, medications, and yes, environmental toxins."

Chronically ill patients include teeth grinders sleeping with airway obstruction. They often struggle with hypothyroid and/or depleted adrenals depleted and undiagnosed. In such cases, recovery begins with:

- A checkup on their liver and gallbladder, with thyroid support
- An airway checkup to unmask Impaired Mouth Syndrome.
- Epigenetic oral appliance to mitigate pain and support sleep.
- Getting "licensed to thrive", i.e., reforming mouth Style to reduce inflammation.

The smart ways to support your liver are (1) deep sleep for nightly renewal, (2) eat healthy: whole non-GMO unprocessed foods free of tap water additives and industrial toxins and pharmaceutical residues, and (3) eat and sleep well. Can your body use WholeHealth Integration care?

WholeHealth Integration

- "Poor thyroid function is like the engine light in your car turning on—it's an indication to open the hood, investigate the engine, and repair what's wrong. You don't want to just take a drug or a supplement that will make the engine light go off." Dr. Datis Kharrazian, author of *Why Do I Still Have Thyroid Symptoms When My Lab Tests Are Normal?11*

- Teeth grinders and sleep apnea patients are chronically ill from oxygen deprivation. Thyroid-liver-gallbladder support is important along with Holistic Mouth Solutions for full health recovery. Cross referrals between AMDs and functional medicine doctors are needed in such cases.

- "Think of thyroid and adrenals as two horses in a team that are pulling your wagon to make the rest of you work," Dr. Tennant says, offering a brilliant analogy: "The first horse to lie down is the thyroid horse. When that happens, the adrenal horse tries to keep pulling. Thus, as you become hypothyroid, your adrenals 'keep pushing through.' You keep trying to do what you need to with sheer willpower even though your voltage is low because you don't have enough thyroid hormone that works. Eventually the adrenal horse wears out too. Now your wagon isn't going anywhere!"

Chapter 14

Adrenal Exhaustion: The Price of Your Health Disruptors

"The more chronic the illness, the more critical the adrenal response becomes."

~ James L. Wilson, ND, DC, PhD,
Adrenal Fatigue: The 21st Century Stress Syndrome[1]

Mirror, mirror on the wall, what's the greatest stress of them all? Confronting death must be one. With teeth grinding and sleep apnea, your body confronts death similarly EVERY night, except that your cognitive brain cannot recall. But your body has its own accounting system, and it sure can tell the raw deal the next morning.

To survive the night, your body has to fight for its life during sleep to get enough air past the choke zone in the back of your mouth. Instead of resting and renewing, sleep becomes a fight to survive.

Sleeping with a 6-foot tiger (tongue) inside a 3-foot cage (mouth) can drain your "batteries" and deplete your adrenals in no time.

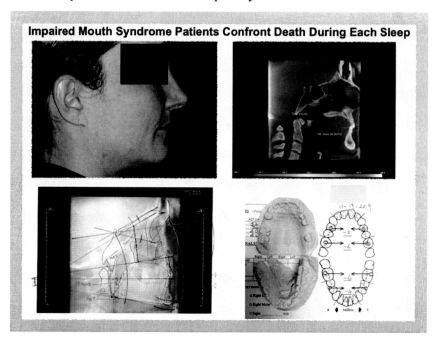

Impaired Mouth Syndrome Patients Confront Death During Each Sleep

Morning fatigue and daytime sleepiness are the price for surviving nightly sleep apnea. You pay the price of poor sleep on waking up: sore jaws, dry mouth, heavy eyelids, groggy mind, and dragging body. Still you push yourself to work at peak performance day after day. Since your sleep is not refreshing you each night, your "gas tank" gradually runs empty over years.

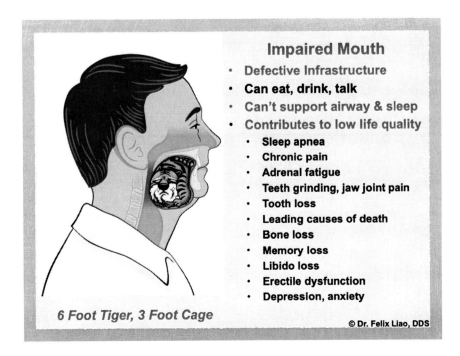

Impaired Mouth
- **Defective Infrastructure**
- **Can eat, drink, talk**
- **Can't support airway & sleep**
- **Contributes to low life quality**
  - **Sleep apnea**
  - **Chronic pain**
  - **Adrenal fatigue**
  - **Teeth grinding, jaw joint pain**
  - **Tooth loss**
  - **Leading causes of death**
  - **Bone loss**
  - **Memory loss**
  - **Libido loss**
  - **Erectile dysfunction**
  - **Depression, anxiety**

6 Foot Tiger, 3 Foot Cage

© Dr. Felix Liao, DDS

As you run on fumes, you compensate for low energy with caffeine or "energy" drinks, sweets like chocolates or candy bars, or crunchy/salty munchies that fuel obesity and inflammation. Exhaustion, collapse, and degenerative diseases are inevitable down that proverbial hill.

"Take it as a general rule that if someone is suffering from a chronic disease and morning fatigue is one of their symptoms, the adrenals are likely involved," writes James L. Wilson, ND, DC, PhD, in *Adrenal Fatigue: The 21st Century Stress Syndrome.*

(Author's note: As used in this book, adrenal fatigue is a symptom description, not a medical diagnosis. A 2016 review[2] concluded "adrenal fatigue does not exist" and "no scientific proof exists to support adrenal fatigue as a true medical condition." Interested readers can search online for hypo-adrenalism or hypo-adrenia to mean low adrenals and use your common sense to judge for yourself.)

It's bad news when your adrenals are down, no matter what the label. Imagine suffering a breakout of hives while on vacation, erectile dysfunction on a romantic get-away, not being able to eat all the goodies at a celebration, or catching a cold with a deadline looming.

Your Adrenal Glands

Biological self-regulation is a built-in ability to keep your body in that narrow zone of balance, a state classically called homeostasis. When you go from lying flat to standing up, it's your adrenals adjusting your circulatory system to gravity so you don't feel lightheaded.

If your self-regulative capacity is strong, you feel well and can recover quickly and uneventfully when accidents/illnesses happen. With poor self-regulation from hypo-thyroid, depleted adrenals, sleep apnea, and health disruptors, you get old and feel old beyond your age, and life becomes a drag.

"The purpose of your adrenal glands is to... enable your body to deal with stress from every possible source, ranging from injury and disease to work and relationship problems," writes Dr. Wilson in *Adrenal Fatigue.*

Adrenaline surges during acute stress such as a fight, a competition, an infection, or threat to life. So, adrenaline is used to treat anaphylaxis, an allergic swelling that can close off the airway. Acute emotional distress or life-threatening trauma/violence can deplete anyone's already overworked adrenals in a flash.

Then there's chronic stress. In the past week, how many times did you find yourself having to "power through"? What do you eat or drink to cope with that challenge? How many years have you been doing this?

Common symptoms of adrenal fatigue, according to Dr. Wilson, can include:

- Insomnia.
- Little or no sex drive.
- Chronic pain and fatigue.
- Susceptibility to allergies.

- Nasal/sinus problems.
- Frequent colds and infections.
- Recurring bronchitis or pneumonia.
- Premenstrual tension.
- Blood sugar swings (a good example of dysregulation, by the way).

The first six are frequently seen in Impaired Mouth Syndrome cases with teeth grinding and sleep apnea patients. In my experience, adrenal fatigue symptoms run rampant among sleep apnea patients, and nearly all doctors and self-employed HCPs suffer from adrenal depletion.

Some people are short-changed on their adrenals. "Children born to mothers already suffering from adrenal fatigue and children who experience severe stress in the womb typically have…less capacity to deal with stress…and so are prone to adrenal fatigue throughout their lives," writes Dr. Wilson.

Chronic illness, health disruptors, bad diet, mental-relationship stress, and staying up late all combine to drain your adrenals. Since teeth grinding is associated with sleep apnea, I suspect adrenal fatigue when I see teeth grinding.

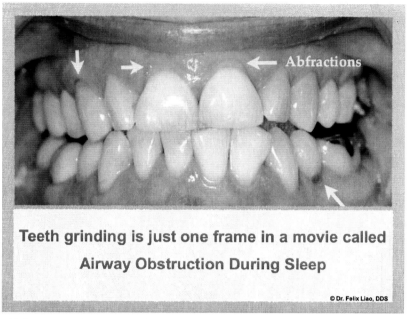

Teeth grinding is just one frame in a movie called
Airway Obstruction During Sleep

© Dr. Felix Liao, DDS

Abfractions (missing a fraction or a piece) are exquisitely sensitive areas of gum recession and root exposure. Abfraction is a result of teeth grinding.

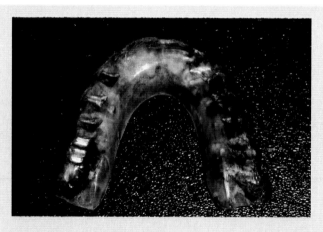

Is this patient still bruxing during sleep?

WHY?

Typical "Night guard" = Missed Opportunity to assess impaired sleep-airway-mouth

© Dr. Felix Liao, DDS

How Your Health Abandons You

When you have frequent colds and infections, your adrenals are likely down. When you get sick and stay sick, it's likely that your adrenals are nearly gone. How did your health slide down that hill?

The graphic below plots adrenal hormones for mobilizing your body to work and fight infections and recover from energy depletion on the vertical axis, so higher is better. The horizontal axis represents the top of health to total failure from left to right.

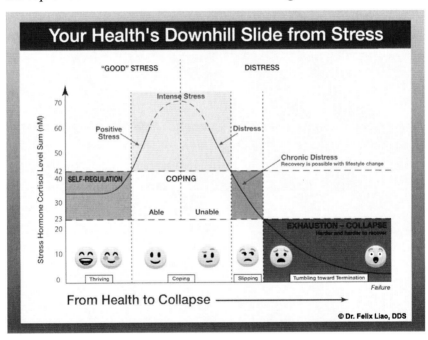

Green Zone: Fully functional adrenals with abundant life force from birth to your college years, when you can handle any stressor with ease.

Yellow Zone: On the up-slope side, your adrenals can handle good stress—pass an exam or go to work. On the downslope, they're not able to keep up and you start having symptoms of adrenal fatigue/depletion.

Orange Zone: The stressors keep coming and health disruptors keep piling up as your adrenals are going down. The compensations—coffee, chocolate, sugar, energy drinks, prescription drugs—aren't working as well. Self-regulation is faltering, which makes you susceptible to Lyme or other infections.

Red Zone: Your adrenals can no longer deal with the sum of health disruptors. This is when you are susceptible to colds and flu progressing to pneumonia, or leaky gut to auto-immune disease like celiac.

How far down the hill is your current state of health? An oral appliance alone is enough on the upper part (yellow box), when the body is not so depleted.

For patients in the orange and red zone, more functional medicine help is needed than epigenetic oral appliance alone. That's where WholeHealth Integration comes in—broken systems are restored back to a functional Whole through out-of-the-box collaboration between mouth doctors, functional medicine and chiropractic doctors, physical, nutritional, myofunctional therapists, and acupuncturists.

How to Recover Your Health with an Empty Tank

Maddy, a 37-year-old, had driven three hours to see me. One look told me that she likely had sleep issues: She had Liao's Sign and dark circles under her eyes. Her hand was ice-cold when we shook hands. I asked her, "Imagine you have a fairy godmother. What symptoms do you put up with every day that you would like her to wave away?"

"I have jaw and facial pain on both sides," she said. "I can't chew. I have nasal congestion all day. I've had neck and back pain for years, despite seeing a chiropractor and massage therapist regularly. I've had four night guards, none of which was helpful."

"Have you been in any car accidents or had surgery or chronic illness?"

"No, but I've had Lyme disease for years, and I'm always exhausted."

At this point, I knew her road to recovery would be a long and bumpy one based on the presence of Liao's Sign, suspected low thyroid function (cold hands), teeth grinding (and poor sleep with it), and a chronic infection (Lyme)—all of which add up to low adrenals.

"You'll need another doctor with expertise in adrenal support, in tandem with oral sleep appliance, to help you recover from your symptoms," I explained. "Just one alone, or the other, won't get you nearly as well as both together—that's what tandem means. Here— take a look at the diagram of your health's downhill slide."

Maddy replied pensively, "I think I'm between the orange and the red zone."

"Oral appliances can help your airway and sleep, but do you understand why you need adrenal support to come back from your Lyme infection, stuffy nose, and aches and pains?"

"Yes, I do now." Maddy's frown turned into a smile. "I have to change my ways and find other doctors to help me."

"That's a *huge* realization and great start. Let me know if you can't find a functional medicine doctor near you, and I'd be glad to make a referral."

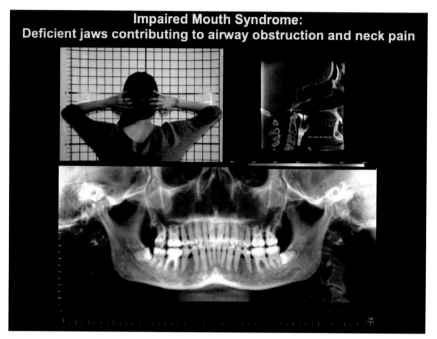

Maddy is pointing to where she has pain all the time.

Principle of Health Keeping and Recovery

Here's how you end up in the red or orange zone: various combinations of overwork, partying, exercising, all the health disruptors, impaired mouth Structure undiagnosed, and impaired mouth Style uncorrected.

The comeback from red-orange to the yellow-green zone is different for each patient, but the principle for recovery never changes. That's to raise energy so your body can self-regulate again to handle stress with greater ease.

Most people overspend their life energy in their youth unknowingly, so they start feeling tired with adrenal depletion as they approach age 40. Many more suffer from airway obstruction and Impaired Mouth Syndrome and sleep apnea undiagnosed. They are on the down slope of the yellow zone in Health's Downhill Slide.

Recovery requires energy to get back uphill. How do you keep going with an empty tank? How do you recover from failing health? This is where you will need good adrenals. Recovery means supporting your adrenals and whole-body health with:

A. Functional thyroid and adrenal hormones
B. Healthy lifestyle following the Chinese Body Clock (chapter 2.4 and 4.4)
C. Holistic mouth Structure to promote deep sleep with wide-open airway
D. Holistic mouth Style to eat to build health and immunity

Which one(s) do you need? You can start with either an AMD (Airway-centered Mouth Doctor®) or Holistic Mouth Consultant—see Afterword.

WholeHealth Integration

♦ Getting your Impaired Mouth Syndrome checked can be a useful first step back from chronic fatigue and illness. In my anecdotal observation, most Lyme disease patients have lower body temperature, Impaired Mouth Syndrome, and adrenal fatigue, making them susceptible to infections and staying ill.

♦ Teeth grinders and sleep apnea patients face death every night during sleep, which can deplete your adrenals faster so you feel older prematurely.

♦ Your energy recovery is not one magic bullet, but a combination of healthy eating and restorative deep sleep (no 6-foot tiger blocking airway), and likely thyroid, adrenal, and other support.

♦ WholeHealth Integration supports functional and sustainable health by:

- Removing health disruptors with functional medicine, nutrition, chiropractics, physical therapy, traditional Chinese medicine, and

- Epigenetic oral appliance to widen jaws and airways to support sleep, and
- Holistic Mouth Style to nourish without overfeeding the body.

Chapter 15

Your Health Destiny: Crash, or Thrive?

"Nature is the source of all true knowledge. She has her own logic, her own laws, she has no effect without cause nor invention without necessity."

~ Leonardo Da Vinci

How will you age—with health and wellness, or pain, misery, and huge medical bills? The key is how well you align your lifestyle with Nature. Your body knows how to run itself, if it has what it needs. This is where you, as the owner-operator, come in again.

What are your greatest fears of growing old? I once did an informal survey with my patients on this question. Their answers: losing my eyesight, my teeth, and my mind.

The big question is *when* you will show up to take charge of your health. It's far too late by the time you have a stroke or come down with Alzheimer's.

Proactive Wellness Care vs. Reactive Disease Management

There are two ways to use your dentist and doctor: as a firefighter or inflammation preventer. Firefighters are critical first responders, but I'd rather not need them.

Root-canal treatment is firefighting reactively. Brushing and flossing is a health-keeping proactively. CPAP and ventilators are reactive. Responding to your body's "early sirens" with Holistic Mouth Solutions is proactive.

The benefits of the proactive approach is summed up in this 2014 MORGEN Study[1] from Europe. Cardiovascular deaths dropped 67% when four traditional lifestyle factors were present: (1) non-smoking, (2) limited alcohol use, (3) 3.5 hours or more of exercise a week, and (4) doing a Mediterranean diet.

When sufficient sleep (7+ hours) was added to the four factors, the risk of cardiovascular death dropped from 67% to 83%. *That* is how to own and operate your mouth proactively.

Reactive medical management has a place. CPAP can serve as a resuscitative device for severe sleep apnea cases with long history and big oxygen debt. If I were in an accident, I'd want the best emergency care at a top trauma hospital, where some operations can solve end-of-the-rope problems. Still, I'd rather not need medical heroics to stay alive. I can stay well and enjoy life by practicing proactive wellness care.

Proactive Wellness Care

It's time to care for your own health rather than depending on your doctors and "health insurance" plans. Your lifestyle is how you use your body, mind, and mouth to live your life. You can't choose your parents or genes, but you can take better care of how you live and eat to build your health.

For example, how many hours a week do you exercise? How much fresh air and outdoor time does your body get each day? How many hours a week do you sit?

Your risk of "type 2 diabetes goes up 91% with high volume sitting time," a 2015 Analysis[2] of 47 studies found. Sitting more than 8 hours a day is high volume.

The same is true for your heart health. "Sitting is associated with all-cause and CVD [cardiovascular disease] mortality risk among the least physically active adults," reports a 2019 Australian study[3]. Your job? "Moderate- to- vigorous physical activity doses equivalent to meeting the current recommendations."

US Center for Disease Control and Prevention[4] states: "The good news is that weight gain can be prevented by choosing a lifestyle that includes good eating habits and daily physical activity."

CDC also says: "By avoiding weight gain, you avoid higher risks of many chronic diseases such as heart disease, stroke, type 2 diabetes, high blood pressure, osteoarthritis, and some forms of cancer."

Holistic Mouth Style specifically supports "good eating habits."

Holistic Mouth Style is the centerpiece of my Proactive Wellness Care that includes:

- Prioritizing Sleep: Wake up refreshed after 7 to 9 hours of sleep.
- Adopting Holistic Mouth Style: Eat foods slowly and mindfully so you can stop at "Just right" to promote health and avoid weight gain.
- Exercising 3.5 hours or more a week as appropriate for your age and health condition.
- Having a strong purpose to live for, not merely eating to exist.
- Balancing work-rest, stress-relaxation, energy demand-recharge, with day-night cycle (see chapter 4).

- Practicing Proactive Self Care to bring out the best in you by:
  - Staying biologically-correct by avoiding known toxins, artificial fragrances, and un-pronounceable ingredients
  - Using natural remedies such as nutrition, digestive supplements, and essential oils to support your body in wellness.

Symptoms like skin itch or joint pain are messages from your body: "Something's wrong here, buddy. I need you to do something." You may not have a say on life's ups and downs, but you *do* control how you respond to your body's messages.

How you respond as owner-CEO of your health determines whether your health goes downhill with side effects or recovers with root-causes corrected. Are you okay with taking drugs to mask bad eating habits? How about shots to mask pain, creams to suppress the itches, or surgery to cut out your body's original parts that have been abused and damaged?

Now, you know there's another way: Proactive Wellness Care. Going forward, diabetes is our main focus as a proactively 100% preventable cause of chronic illness originating from impaired mouth style and lifestyle.

Diabetes and Metabolic Syndrome Come from Impaired Mouth Style

Diabetes was the seventh largest cause of death in 2015, says CDC[5]: "Average medical expenditures for people with diagnosed diabetes were about $13,700 per year." That is "about 2.3 times higher than the same age and sex without diabetes."

Diabetes Fast Facts	Prediabetes Fast Facts
• **Total:** 30.3 million people have diabetes (9.4% of the US population) • **Diagnosed:** 23.1 million people • **Undiagnosed:** 7.2 million people (23.8% of people with diabetes are undiagnosed)	• **Total:** 84.1 million adults aged 18 years or older have prediabetes (33.9% of the adult US population) • **65 years or older:** 23.1 million adults aged 65 years or older have prediabetes

Fast Facts Source: *U.S. Center For Disease Control and Prevention*

Why so much higher? Diabetes comes with a long list of complications per American Diabetes Association[6]:

- Skin: itching, fungal and bacterial infections, blisters, and other eruptions
- Eyes: cataracts, glaucoma, retinopathy
- Neuropathy: about half of all diabetics have some nerve damage
- Feet: tingling, numbness, weakness, infections, ulcerations, gangrene, amputation
- High blood pressure
- Stroke: 1.5 times greater risk of brain damage from ruptured artery
- Kidney disease: often without symptoms until total failure strikes

The horses have long left the barn by the time vision loss, stroke, neuropathy, and kidney damage is/are diagnosed. WHO has been attending to your barn?

Smart owner-operators will focus on what comes before diabetes: metabolic syndrome (MetS)—a cluster of conditions that can raise your risk of heart disease and stroke—as well as diabetes. A large waistline is a visible sign of metabolic syndrome. Others include high triglycerides, low LDL ("good") cholesterol, high blood pressure, and high fasting blood sugar.

How do you avoid it? One way is to monitor your blood sugar at home. Being mindful of each mouthful is another. A potbelly stems from a runaway mouth.

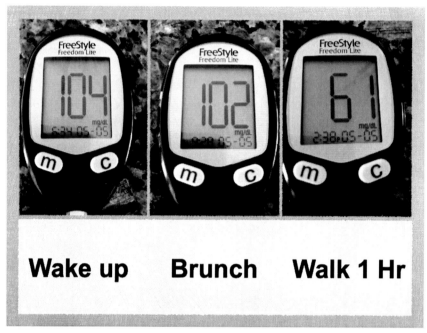

Monitoring your blood sugar is a powerful motivator to exercise, which is among the recommended ways to lower diabetes risk along with knowing how to eat for health.

Slow Down Your Eating

Fast eaters were 59% more likely than slow eaters to get high triglyceride which contributes to hardening of arteries, found a 2019 study from Spain[7].

A 2019 study from Japan[8] likewise found slow eating can help prevent metabolic syndrome: "Participants with 0-9 teeth who ate quickly had a significantly higher [statistical risk] for MetS compared with those with 20-28 teeth who ate slowly." That's one more reason that dentists-turned-mouth-doctors are well-suited to deliver proactive wellness care.

Making a Declaration to Thrive

Declaration to Thrive is your mission statement on how you will use your mouth and live your life. It's your North Star to guide your health behavior.

For myself, I want to live to age 100 with every system in my body working and nothing hurting or limiting. Then, I'm open to renegotiating my deal with God. Given my age and history, here's what I have to do to thrive:

A. Get my mouth structurally sound to support sleep with wide-open airway (next slide).

B. Align with WholeHealth doctors and healthcare professionals (chapter 1).

C. Get "licensed to thrive" with a health-building mouth Style to build health and enjoy life (chapters 4 and 5).

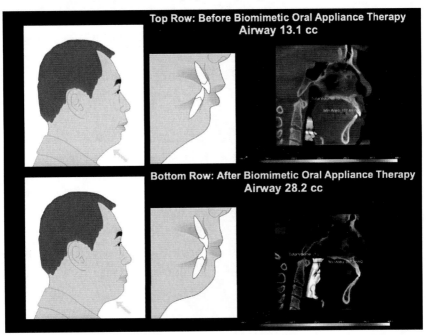

Above: CT images above show the before and after results of epigenetic oral appliance therapy. Airway volume more than doubled, and the new airway is wide (all white) without a choke zone.

Below: My sleep test score below is at 6.1 from 23 after epigenetic oral appliances.

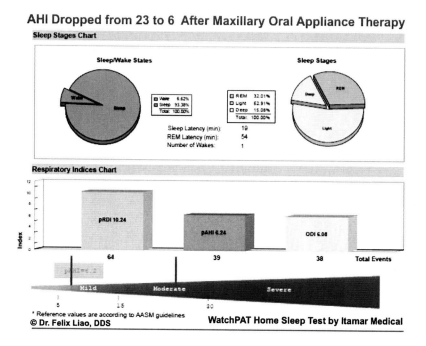

AHI Dropped from 23 to 6 After Maxillary Oral Appliance Therapy

What's your Declaration to Thrive? Take a minute to reflect and write it down. (If you don't write it, it doesn't stick.) If you're coming up blank, you can borrow mine for now and then customize it later. This Declaration to Thrive clarifies how you want to end up and therefore how to get there.

WholeHealth Integration

♦ Holistic Mouth Style is the centerpiece of Proactive Wellness Care that's 100% in your control. Slow down to eat without rushing so your gut can signal your brain that it is truly ready to eat, or to stop.

♦ You may not have a say on life's ups and downs, but you DO have 100% control of how you respond to your body's messages and whether your symptoms get managed with side effects or resolved at root-cause level.

- Without your Declaration to Thrive, you are more likely to end up at the bottom of health's downhill slide with an empty tank. With it as your GPS, you can stop wilting and start thriving.

Chapter 16

Stop Wilting:
4 Keys to Start Thriving

"An unexamined life is not worth living."

~ Socrates

Your mouth is the gateway into your body, and the only part of your digestive system where you have 100% control. How well is it working?

A Holistic Mouth is structurally sound and sensibly used to support whole-body health. Alignment, Breathing, Circulation, and Digestion (ABCD) are the 4 keys of Proactive Wellness Care for vibrant health. All too often, they are missing in the care of health.

Consider the presenting complaints of the following new patients I saw in a single week. They all have seen their own doctors and dentists for years. Ask yourself what's missing in their ABCD:

GK, male, age 66: brain fog and poor concentration since age 8; fear and depression; low energy and stamina; constipation-diarrhea; trouble with initiating urination and bladder emptying from prostate enlargement; voice becoming more hoarse; strong sweet tooth.

DJ, female, age 45: too many broken teeth ("I have terrible teeth grinding," she explained, "and a loose tooth that's painful to touch now"); right knee pain; neck pain with herniated disks; spacing out mid-sentence. DJ had a history of car accidents. Gastric bypass surgery had helped her reduce from 320 to 180 pounds. "Emotional eating" had led to her runaway weight.

TMG, male, age 46: lack of self-confidence due to the appearance of his open bite; low back pain for 20 years and getting worse; daily anxiety and adrenal fatigue starting around 1 p.m. followed by a crash at 3; snoring, teeth grinding, and waking up with jaws clenched; Lyme disease from a tick bite 11 years prior.

FY, male, age 55: low back pain every day for 15 to 20 years and getting worse, limiting exercise; nightmares and waking with an "I can't breathe!" sensation; chronic sinusitis impacted by diet, made worse with cheese and sugar, better with low carb; he is a pilot who has managed his sleep apnea with mandibular advancement appliances and wants to avoid CPAP.

CJ, female, age 68: partial facial paralysis for 14 years that started with a trip and falling on her forehead, resulting in two stitches and lots of neck problems ever since; crushing fatigue when she "runs out of gas"; severe benign positional vertigo that began with a failed compost toilet and septic water under her kitchen floor; recent acute stress related to her angry mother dying of Alzheimer's and sister with lung cancer at the same time. The image below shows her 3-foot cage and head-jaws-neck misalignment.

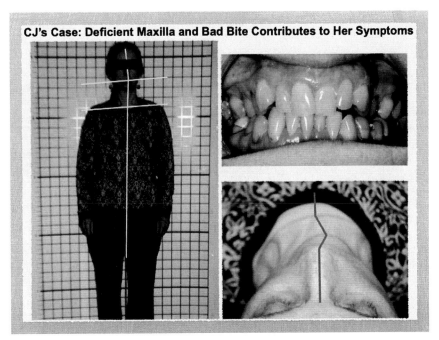

CJ's Case: Deficient Maxilla and Bad Bite Contributes to Her Symptoms

CJ's dentist was trained to see and fix teeth and gums, not Impaired Mouth Syndrome.

SK, female, age 30: teeth grinding; snoring; bad migraines around eyes (some improvement with gluten-free diet); aches and pains in neck, shoulders, and back; weak mid-face and weak chin after braces in high school and clear aligners. Her airway volume (shown in the next slide) was just under 50% of low comfort. She wants to start a family: "I'm hoping to start a family next year." She gets that an optimal maternal airway is crucial for her new child and decides to take the proactive step to start epigenetic oral appliance therapy.

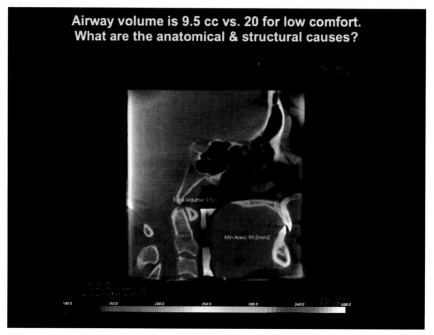

Upgrading maternal airway can better support a baby toward fuller genetic potential.

Where do you start?

Limited clinical outcome and patient frustration can come from silo mentality when each profession is locked into its own "standard of care" without seeing the whole patient and without knowing what others can do.

Putting the patient back together takes more than fixing local symptoms. Health recovery and up-building takes *integration* of *all* systems. Since the mouth is to humans what roots are to plants, WholeHealth Integration starts with wide-open airway to deliver oxygen during sleep and eating right to build health and empower immunity.

Four Keys to Start Thriving

If your body is a garden, then what does your health need from you, the gardener, to thrive? Be sure to address four key functions, best in the ABCD order: Alignment, Breathing, Circulation, and Digestion.

And yes, ABCD comes before dental implants, orthodontics, cosmetics, or reconstructions. The only exception is dental infection control to clean up cavities, bleeding gums, and root-canal infections and jaw cavitation.

Alignment is first because health needs structure (form) to perform functions. Gravity never stops pulling us toward the grave; thus, proper alignment is a requirement for nerve and blood supply. Pinched nerves cause pain, and artery narrowing makes heart disease. Conversely, choked airway widens when jaws are treated epigenetically to their genetic potential: room for all 28 teeth to line up straight (wisdom teeth excepted in adults). Chronic head-neck-back pain often goes away when the lower jaw can fit into the upper without a hitch in the jaw joints. Alignment of mouth Structure is a pre-requisite of a functional airway.

Breathing starts with nasal function and structure. Snoring is mouth breathing during sleep. Teeth grinding means your body is confronting death and doing CPR on itself in response to airway obstruction. The tongue must occupy the airway if the jaws are underdeveloped for all your teeth. Sleep is not a time to fend off death from oxygen deprivation, but renewal time to recharge your batteries and repair your daily wear and tear.

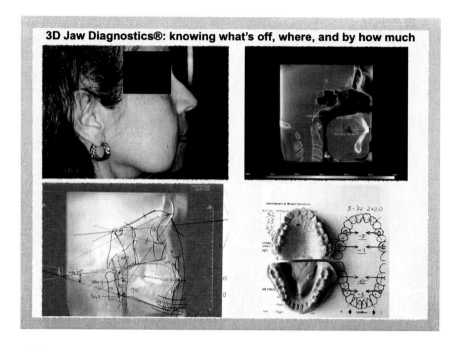

3D Jaw Diagnostics®: knowing what's off, where, and by how much

This patient had just finished 2 years of braces. Her presenting symptoms include chronic pain, fatigue, airway, teeth grinding, and more. 3D Jaw Diagnostics® helps custom design an oral appliance to target what's off and where in the "3-foot cage."

Circulation should deliver oxygen and nutrients, not infections and toxins. See a biological dentist to rule out oral infections and a physician to rule out any respiratory, digestive, urinary, or skin infections. Sleep apnea overworks your heart, and oxygen deficiency grows bad bacteria—just two more reasons to first get an airway checkup with an Airway-centered Mouth Doctor® (AMD).

Digestion gets you energy from food to build health and maintain your body. Digestion starts with your mouth where you have 100% control. The point of eating is not congestion, obesity, or inflammation. This means training yourself on how to eat right, which is the point of holistic mouth Style. You can do this by yourself or under the guidance of your healthcare professional of choice.

WholeHealth Integration is a platform where functional medicine, body work, nutrition, and all therapy modalities of the East and West can work with AMDs to put each patient back to a functional whole, starting with ABCD.

If impaired mouth structure is a hidden source of so many medical-dental-mood symptoms, then what's its root cause? Given how widespread Impaired Mouth Syndrome is, it's good to know the answer for proactive wellness care.

Tracing the footprints from the crime scene to the perpetrator, you'd find either a tongue-tie or a stuffy nose, or both. Until very recently, this form and function awareness was largely missing in doctors' practices and parental awareness.

Origin of Impaired Mouth Structure

What contributes to teeth crowding, jaw underdevelopment, and misalignment?

The answers are many, including but not limited to the standard American diet (SAD) high in additives and low in growth factors, habitual mouth breathing, improper weaning, health disruptors listed in the last 3 chapters, and tongue-tie.

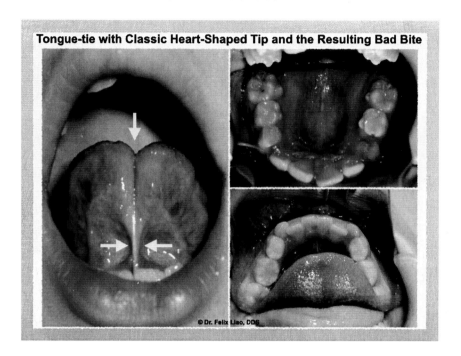

Tongue-tie with Classic Heart-Shaped Tip and the Resulting Bad Bite

A severe tongue-tie can impair breastfeeding to distress both the newborn and mom. A less obvious but nonetheless disempowering tongue-tie, however, often goes unnoticed in dental checkups. This can result in the wrong arch getting the stimulation from the tongue for extra-development.

Alignment in the dental-facial skeleton is correct when maxilla (upper) arch is wider for the mandible (lower) arch to fit into, like a shoe for your foot. Which one needs to be bigger? Breastfeeding facilitates this orthopedically-correct alignment. The maxilla develops preferentially from two sources: (1) nasal breathing, and (2) tongue milking the nipple against the palate.

A tongue-tie anchors the tongue to the floor of the mouth, thereby not stimulating the upper jaw to be larger (the shoe) for the lower jaw (the foot) to fit into without strain. The resulting discrepancy (smaller maxilla larger mandible) often entraps the mandible, drives the tongue deeper into the airway, and throws off the neck spine—creating pain and Impaired Mouth Syndrome.

A Dentist's Journey from Tongue-Tie to Airway

"Dear Dr. Liao, I came to see you after 4 months of numb fingers on both hands. You said I was tongue-tied and it could be connected to my numb fingers. It surprised me but made total sense. My MRI and neurologist had said my numb fingers were coming from stenosis [narrowing] on C6, C7, C8," Dr. RL emailed me a year later.

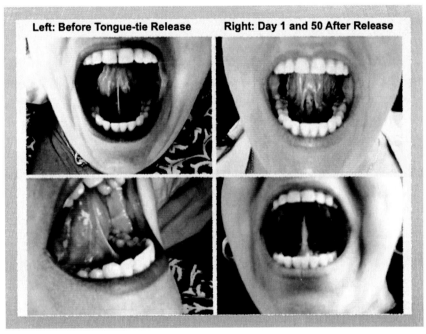

The tongue-tie case of Dr. RL. The lower left image in the slide below shows a "Cave Maneuver" to reprogram the tongue to stay in touch with the palate, where it belongs, instead of the floor of the mouth.

She continued: "After your gracious consult, I started to use a simple appliance to guide my tongue into its correct position, and when I wore the appliance the numbness would disappear—that confirmed your view that the tongue tie was related and I felt that releasing the tongue was much less aggressive compared to neck surgery.

"A month after meeting you, I bought a laser, then I spent a day with Dr. Richard Baxter in Tennessee and watched him release lots of kids. He released my tongue at the end of that day and my numb fingers went away immediately.

"I can't thank you enough for opening my eyes to my tongue tie. My entire life I would get massages twice a month and told them to spend 90 minutes on just my neck and shoulders. Since I was released my neck and shoulders have been 100% stress-free. It's amazing no tension at all. This release has been the greatest gift ever and I owe it all to you so [t]hank you!"

I am so proud of Dr. RL for making the necessary investment and training to help patients with tongue-tie release and more: "It is the most rewarding procedure out of everything I do. I've since became certified as an oral myologist [to provide myofunctional therapy]."

Oral-facial myofunctional therapy (OMT) is physical therapy for the mouth and surrounding facial tissues. It trains the tongue, lips, and cheeks to swallow correctly 1,500 times a day and to achieve lip seal to promote optimal dental-facial development in children, avoiding relapse of front-teeth crowding in adults after oral appliance therapy.

OMT also supports sleep apnea by toning the flaccid muscles in the back of the mouth and throat. "Myofunctional therapy decreases apnea-hypopnea index [sleep apnea score] by approximately 50% in adults and 62% in children," reports this 2015 study[1]. Breathing and sleeping well is well worth your effort.

Upon tongue-tie release, patients often feel a loosening of their entire body, in my experience. One career navy man had tears running down his cheeks right after his tongue-tie release: "I can finally breathe without restriction for the first time in my life." Anatomically, the floor of the mouth is connected by fascia (soft skeleton) through the neck vertebrae down the breastbone to the heart and lung sacs, and the nerves to the fingers originate in the neck.

Connecting these dots, you can see why Dr. RL's numb fingers went away with tongue-tie release: "I learned after 27 years of dentistry that the neck and shoulder tension was not just a result of my chosen profession but also a result of my tongue tie all life long." She's learned WholeHealth Integration firsthand.

WholeHealth Integration means putting the patient back together into a functional Whole. It starts with ruling out impaired mouth Structure (in all its hard and soft tissues) before invasive neck surgery, endless massage therapy, or life-long dependence on a machine.

WholeHealth Integration

- The mouth is a critical infrastructure for airway, sleep, and freedom from chronic fatigue and pain. If you are living with Impaired Mouth Syndrome undiagnosed, your health and wellness care will fall short.

- Alignment and Airway must be addressed before standard dentistry, including braces, implants, cosmetic and reconstructive work, to avoid unnecessary complications and cost.

- Behind every impaired mouth Structure lurks a tongue-tie, stuffy nose, or both. Myofunctional therapy with tongue-tie release can be a powerful part of Holistic Mouth Solutions.

- Sleep apnea patients with CPAP intolerance have an oral appliance option. See a qualified AMD to get your airway imaged, get a sleep test if indicated, and find a treatment that matches your healthcare values.

Chapter 17

Why Alignment and Airway First

You see only what you know,
hence you can't diagnose what you don't know.

~ Dr. Richard Beistle, DDS

None of us could hold up our own head at birth, but we all could suckle for dear life. Our growth and development start from the mouth downward. The foundation of our body is not the feet but the head and the jaws.

That's why jaw under-development spells health trouble throughout the body. Impaired Mouth Syndrome means impaired head functions. As this 2012 study[1] concludes, "Pediatric obstructive sleep apnea in non-obese children is a disorder of oral-facial growth."

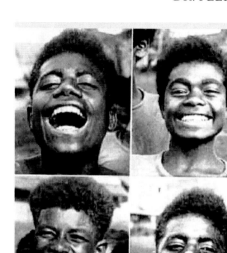

Natural Wellness

Full genetic potential looks and works like this:

- **Broad** faces
- **Wide** arches
- **Balanced** head and jaws
- **High cheekbones**
- **Radiant health**
- **Spontaneous joy**
- **No need for pediatricians**
- **No need for braces**

Images Courtesy of Sally Fallon, Weston A. Price Foundation.

These faces in the slide above captured by Dr. Weston A. Price serve as my "North Star" in redeveloping "3-foot cage" with epigenetic oral appliances. Full genetic potential means enough upper and lower jawbone volume for all 32 natural teeth to line up straight, regardless of each patient's ethnic background.

Dentally, deficient jaws that don't grow to their full potential come with crooked teeth, malocclusion (bad bite is good only for pain), teeth grinding, and lots of failed dental work despite brushing. Medically, underdeveloped jaws are literally a pain in the neck going down the back to hips and knees. They also mean a narrow airway, oxygen deprivation, and persistent symptoms that defy conventional treatment.

The Teeth Tell the Tale!

STRAIGHT TEETH WIDE Dental Arches	CROOKED, CROWDED TEETH Narrow Dental Arches
Plenty of room in head for pituitary, pineal, hypothalamus	Compromised space for master glands in the head
Good skeletal development, good muscles	Poor development, poor posture, easily injured
Keen eyesight and hearing	Poor eyesight and hearing
Optimal function of all organs	Compromised function of all organs
Optimistic outlook, learns easily	Depression, behavior problems, learning problems
Round pelvic opening, easy childbirth	Oval pelvic opening, difficult childbirth

Slide Courtesy of Sally Fallon, WAP Foundation

The good news is, deficient jaws can now be redeveloped without pain and regardless of age, provided you have healthy natural teeth.

Jaw Redevelopment Can Fix Pain Naturally

In healthy development, the airway in the back of your mouth widens as the jaws grow. Correctly designed to target what's off, epigenetic oral appliances can redevelop both jaws, widen your oral airway, plus fix aches and pains stemming from the "3-foot cage."

More than 95% of my cases start with alignment and airway to support breathing and circulation. The exceptions are (1) dental fires (cavities and infected root-canals) to be extinguished or (2) CPAP for urgent rescue.

With epigenetic redevelopment of the maxilla comes pain mitigation or resolution in, around, and far beyond the mouth—something other ways of treating sleep apnea can't deliver. When the mandible can fit comfortably into the maxilla without strain, many cases of neck-shoulder-back pain go away without return. It's like removing a thorn from the foot and walking can be normal again, only this thorn is jaw misalignment.

Additional thorns can include whiplash from accidents, traumatic blows, surgical screws or scars, medical factors, and/or "extraction and retraction" orthodontics to straighten teeth without regard to alignment and airway. This next case involves a patient who had eaten healthy and done yoga for years and a history of subtraction orthodontics in his teens—4 adult teeth pulled and the resulting spaces closed with braces.

'My Healthcare Home Run'

"I'm here for a second opinion on implants," said Brian M. at his first visit with me. "I had a root-canal done, and I don't want another one after Googling 'root canal toxicity.' And I don't want any metals in my mouth either. I know all about galvanic currents from dental metals."

"I love meeting fellow engineers—always so sound in logic!" I said, shaking his hand (it was pre-COVID-19). His hand was cold. I also noticed Liao's Sign in his facial profile, suggesting airway obstruction. I then started my evaluation.

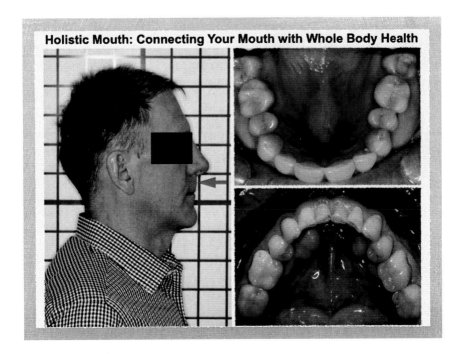

Holistic Mouth: Connecting Your Mouth with Whole Body Health

"I see you keep a spotlessly clean mouth," I said. Tooth #27—his lower right cuspid—had a root-canal treatment but no filling before. "Do you recall any trauma to this tooth? A blow or whiplash accident?" He didn't, so I shared my suspicion that his airway was the issue. "Grinding to try to keep your airway open can kill your tooth from oxygen deprivation to its nerve."

"I read about that already in *Early Sirens*." He grinned. "I just wanted to hear you say it as the author. So, what can be done?"

"I see you had four teeth extracted when you had braces done. Did your tongue get trimmed with the extractions so it could still fit in the smaller cage resulting?"

"No," he chuckled, "but I get it. After they closed the spaces with braces, I wound up with a six-foot tiger in a two-foot cage."

"You'd have made a great mouth doctor," I told him. "So, what are the three symptoms you'd most like your fairy godmother to wave away?"

"That's easy," he said. "For one, that root-canaled tooth is still sore after a year. I'd like it to not be. Plus, I've got nasal congestion, wake up to pee three or four times every night, and have low testosterone symptoms."

"I don't diagnose or treat any medical conditions, but I do see how your structurally impaired mouth is likely contributing to your issues."

"I'm ready to start! Let's get rid of the root cause that killed my tooth #27 so no other tooth suffers the same fate."

I then referred him to an endodontist to get the tooth retreated with new technology and fitted him with an epigenetic oral appliance to redevelop his super-deficient lower jaw.

"After we finish that redevelopment," I assured him, "you can do whatever you want with that tooth." Brian's curiosity about dental implants fell by the wayside upon realizing the importance of addressing the more fundamental issues of alignment and airway.

Brian has since called his epigenetic oral appliance a "healthcare home run." He says that it fixed his lower back pain, improved his yoga, deepened his sleep, and gave him far more energy. "I didn't expect that fixing my jaws and airway would also fix all that. My mouth (from extraction-retraction orthodontics) was where I was stuck, and I was not moving forward no matter what else I did until this piece of a complex puzzle was fixed," he said. "And, by the way, my knee pain is also gone." See Resources for links to Brian M's and others' video testimonials.

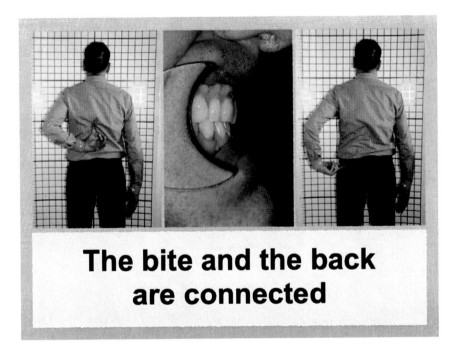

The bite and the back are connected

Once the jaws are orthopedically aligned and the airway is enlarged, the whole body can finally relax. The most frequent feedback I get from patients who start epigenetic jaw redevelopment include: aches and pains go away and do not return; chiropractic adjustment holds longer; mood and brain fog lift; food intolerance improves; and the mask of fatigue is replaced by a pinkish facial glow.

Dental Implants: Only After ABCD

Every part of the body needs Alignment, Breathing, Circulation and Digestion. This is true for natural teeth and dental implants alike. You don't want dental implants to fail not only because of the pain and cost, but also because nothing is available next.

If grinding is damaging to natural teeth, it is fatal to dental implants. Teeth grinders had 3.3 times greater implant failures compared to non-grinders, found this 2016 study[2] of 2670 patients with over 10,000 total implants.

By contrast, teeth grinding stopped in sleep apnea patients whose CPAP is properly titrated during sleep test, reported this 2002 study[3]. So, opening airway obstruction solves teeth grinding.

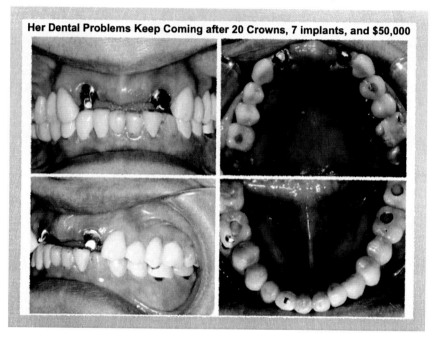

Her Dental Problems Keep Coming after 20 Crowns, 7 implants, and $50,000

In the slide above, the patient's upper front replacement teeth fell out for the third time. Nearly every tooth in her mouth had been treated at considerable cost. The result is frustrating to both the patient and the dentist, who is a victim of the "dentists do teeth" silo mentality.

All this dental work shows up in her panoramic dental X-ray below—and just below that, CT imaging shows her super-choked airway. That airway—in the red-to-black zone—had never been part of her dental evaluation. Also note the screw from her neck spine surgery, showing up bright white near the lower edge of the lower left image. Her neck pain was bad enough to require surgery. Impaired mouth structure likely contributed to her neck pain, in my opinion.

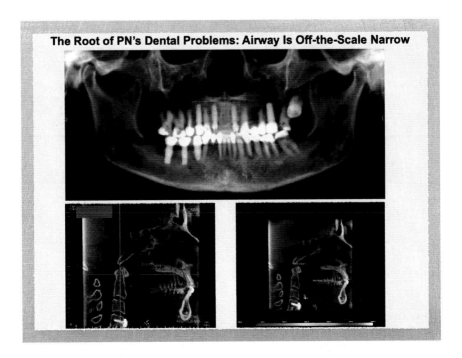

The Root of PN's Dental Problems: Airway Is Off-the-Scale Narrow

Silo mentality is the prevailing norm in dentistry in 2020s America. Fortunately, dentists are starting to see the need for airway diagnosis and WholeHealth integration. If only more healthcare professionals could buy into Alignment and Airway as a foundation for healthier circulation and digestion.

If you wish to avoid costly mistakes, then do dental implants and new teeth and braces only **after** ABCD is met. The nerve tissues inside your own teeth need ABCD to stay alive too. Doing reconstructive dental work, or aligning teeth with braces, without considering ABCD amounts to re-arranging furniture inside a collapsing house.

'I'm so glad there's hope now for my teeth.'

Angie, a trim 40-year-old athletic trainer, came to see me after becoming aware of her "violent teeth grinding"—a complaint made by her ex-partner. She reported waking up tired four or five days every week since her college years; daytime sleepiness; super sensitivity to noise; and fatigue. She had lost two teeth already and now had a loose root-canaled tooth. She was teary-eyed as she told me how desperately she wanted to save the rest of her teeth.

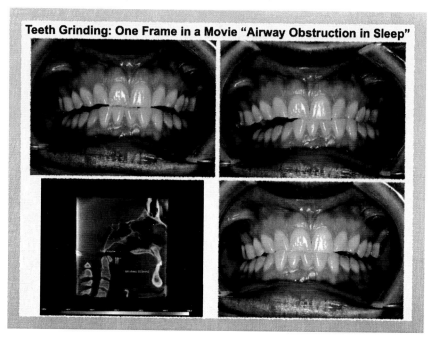

Teeth Grinding: One Frame in a Movie "Airway Obstruction in Sleep"

We talked about ABCD and how grinding is a telltale sign of a compromised airway; likewise, her sleepiness and fatigue. "It makes perfect sense," she said. "None of the five night guards I've had made any real difference. They were uncomfortable, and I just kept grinding anyway."

"I'm not surprised. Dentists are taught night guards because their professors did not know what else to do for teeth grinding. Teeth grinding is rooted in airway obstruction—that's a new discovery with the advent of sleep medicine and CT technology. Your airway obstruction is so severe that it's a miracle you're still alive!"

The upper right image in the slide below shows her airway was in the red-black (extremely choked) zone, and the upper left shows where her pain is.

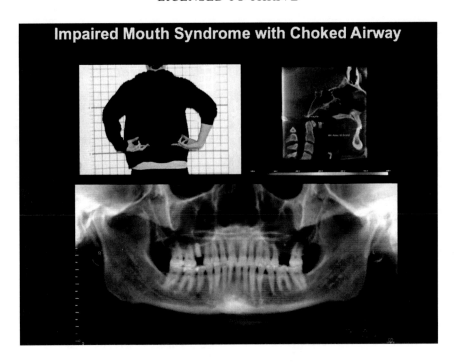

Impaired Mouth Syndrome with Choked Airway

"I know that now after reading *Early Sirens*. Before, I had asked my dentist what we could do about my narrow airway. He said, 'Nothing.' I'm so glad there's hope now for me and the rest of my teeth!"

My heart goes out to Angie, as well as her dentist—another victim of the traditional "in the box" mindset, limiting their power to help heal dental patients.

Angie's 2-month update said: "I'm happy to report I do feel I am breathing better already. Mostly it feels like my nasal passages have opened some. The weekly expansion has been relatively easy. My body seems to be adapting and adjusting well. Altogether, it's been wonderful…already a relief and I'm grateful."

Case Study of Another Dentist

Like their patients, dentists and indeed all healthcare professionals are not immune from Impaired Mouth Syndrome. Dr. RK is a general dentist who took up training with me to become an Airway

Mouth Doctor® (AMD) way back in 2017. Based on her Liao's Sign and the CT image of her airway, I recommended a sleep test. The threshold for severe apnea is 30 AHI. She scored 37.

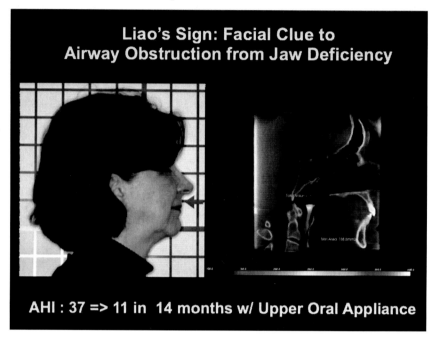

Liao's Sign: Facial Clue to Airway Obstruction from Jaw Deficiency

AHI : 37 => 11 in 14 months w/ Upper Oral Appliance

Dr. RK had sustained a rotator cuff injury while being pulled out of the birth canal, but despite one surgery and repeated physical therapy, she never could raise her dominant hand above her ear. Her hand and fingers weren't affected, though. She went through college, dental school, and practiced dentistry for 25 years that way.

Before starting her AMD training, Dr. RK had actually taken a sleep test before, which scored her AHI at 68. "I started on CPAP right away, and I consider myself a CPAP success story," she said. "Once I recovered from a lifetime of sleep deprivation, my hormones started to regulate—cortisol, ghrelin, and leptin. The next year, I started yet another weight loss and wellness program, but this time I lost 110 pounds. I'd never been able to keep weight off before."

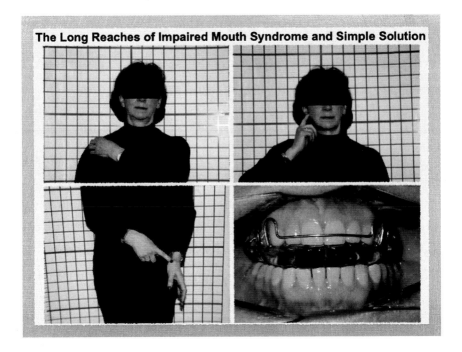

The Long Reaches of Impaired Mouth Syndrome and Simple Solution

But her impaired mouth Structure remains untouched by CPAP. Recall that Alignment comes before Airway and Breathing? Dr. RK admitted, "I've had orthodontics three times in my life, twice as an adult, but none of the orthodontists looked at my airway anatomy." It was time for a Holistic Mouth Solution.

Once we started epigenetic oral appliance therapy, Dr. RK's AHI dropped from 37 to 11 (mild) in 14 months. And just look what it did for her right shoulder:

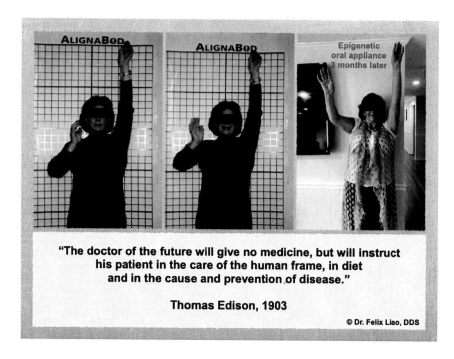

"The doctor of the future will give no medicine, but will instruct his patient in the care of the human frame, in diet and in the cause and prevention of disease."

Thomas Edison, 1903

© Dr. Felix Liao, DDS

Could I have predicted this outcome? No. But now we know better from this precedent.

"Why doesn't my chiropractic adjustments hold?!" Patients often ask in frustration. "Why does my neck-shoulder pain come back in a few days?" The short answer: Impaired mouth structure needs to be treated at the same time.

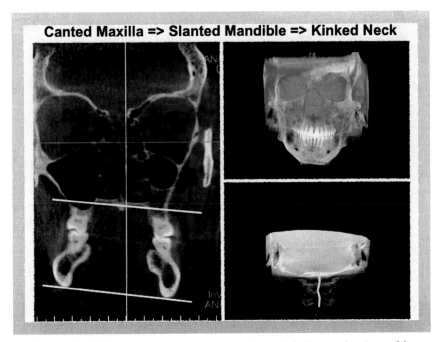

Above: Dr. RK's upper jaw was canted high left (green line), and her lower jaw (yellow line) and neck (blue line) had no chance of being aligned.

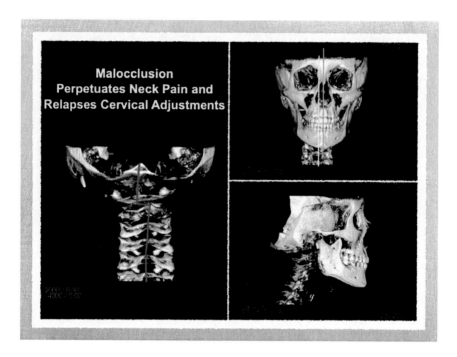

Retruded jaws and dental midlines being off leads, predictably, to neck-shoulders-back pain and misaligned neck vertebrae, in my experience. Said pain often goes away either fully or substantially when the jaws are redeveloped and the bite realigned. Car accidents and traumatic blows to the jaws are other aggravators. If and when chiropractic adjustments do not hold consistently, see a trained AMD to rule out Impaired Mouth Syndrome as a perpetuator of recurring pain.

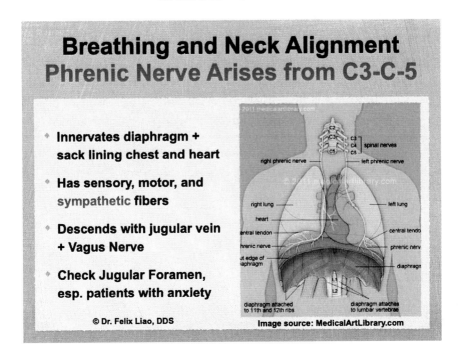

The phrenic nerve supplying the diaphragm arises from neck spine segments C3-5, which is often thrown off by impaired mouth structure, in my experience.

The jaws-neck-shoulders-back are connected, so are jaws and airway—that common sense is regularly lacking in the experience of patients who come to see me. It's time for all healthcare professionals to adopt Alignment and Airway first to promote restorative sleep and uninterrupted oxygen supply as the first requirements to survival and thriving wellness.

WholeHealth Integration

- Recovering your health, including losing weight and keeping it off, is easier and more sustainable with Impaired Mouth Structure (and associated airway obstruction) diagnosed and sleep improved with airway widening.

- Airway obstruction is rooted in impaired mouth structure, which should have first-line consideration in WholeHealth Integration.

- Unblocking airway obstruction stops teeth grinding. Missing this point can be very expensive if dental implants and cosmetic dentistry are done without observing Alignment, Breathing, Circulation, and Digestion first.

- Wherever you have recurring medical, dental, mood, and/or pain symptoms, look "upstream"—it's safer to assume there's an oral contribution than to ignore or dismiss it.

Chapter 18

Nosing Your Way to Holistic Mouth Solutions

"How you breathe as a child determines how you look the rest of your life."

~ Patrick McKeown,
Shut Your Mouth and Change Your Life[1]

A good-looking face, high cheekbones, beautiful jaw lines, and full-throated wellness come as a package when both jaws are fully developed to their genetic potential. Inside this well-formed structure are functional spaces to carry out important health functions, including alignment, airway, breathing, eating, swallowing, and speaking.

Upper Airway Functional Spaces

- **Zone 1: Nasal Cavity**

- **Zone 2: Nasal Pharynx**

- **Zone 3: Oral Pharynx**

- **Zone 4: Oral Cavity**

- **Functional upper airway: ALL 4 zones are wide open.**

- **Airway-centered Mouth Doctor® is the diagnostician and the wellness architect.**

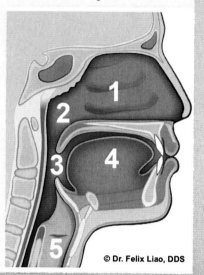

© Dr. Felix Liao, DDS

Breathing begins with Zone 1; that's why my new patient evaluation starts with listening to and observing for nasal obstruction. Dental checkup comes last. Thriving health requires a wide-open upper airway in *all* 4 zones.

Narrowing in just one zone means breathing dysfunction and susceptibility to respiratory issues. Because the maxilla occupies the mid-face and provides the floor and walls of the nasal passage and sinuses, its deficient development often means narrower Zones 1, 2, and 3.

Optimal dental-facial development starts with nasal breathing and lip seal. In children, long-term mouth breathing can lead to a long and narrow "horsey" face, lackluster appearance, crooked and jumbled teeth, frequent respiratory infections, and a greater risk of relapse after braces.

"All mouth breathers have crooked teeth," says leading Buteyko Breathing instructor Patrick McKeown[1]. "Straight teeth do not create a good-looking face, but a good face creates straight teeth."

I agree totally—good faces come from fully developed jaws with room for all teeth to line up straight.

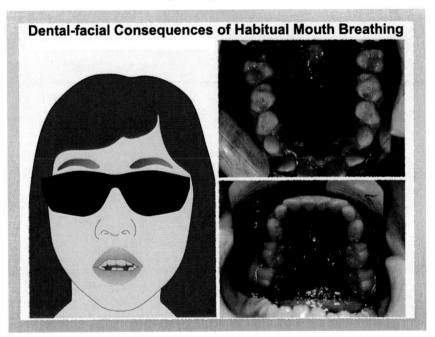

Dental-facial Consequences of Habitual Mouth Breathing

An extreme case of mouth breathing from nasal obstruction undiagnosed for too long.

Nasal, sinus, and throat symptoms and snoring are common in adults with sleep apnea, chronic pain, and fatigue. They often grew up with mouth breathing unnoticed or had subtraction orthodontics (extraction of adult teeth and spaces closed with braces). The result is impaired mouth structure, continued stuffy nose, or frequently both. A chairside chat then follows on the need to change their mouth Structure and Style.

Snoring is mouth breathing from nasal blockage during sleep. Snoring is a health risk, not just an annoyance to your sleep partner, especially with daytime sleepiness. Heavy snoring (4 or more nights a week) comes with twice the risk for diabetes[2] and stroke[3]—and both carry serious consequences.

Nasal Obstructors

Habitual mouth breathing from stuffy nose brings on many problems: chapped lips, a dry tongue, bleeding gums, dragon breath, swollen tonsils, tiredness, more colds and flu, and a down-and-out appearance. So, what causes nasal obstruction?

Take a moment to think about the foods you commonly consume and activities you engage in regularly. Which of the following show up on your list?

- Food: eggs, cheese, bread, dairy products, pasta, soy, corn, oats
- Drinks: water, fruit juices, alcohol (beer and wine), soft drinks, sport drinks
- Snacks: cakes, pies, cookies, ice cream, candies, chips and dips, fries, nuts
- Substances: sugar, salt, caffeine, alcohol, tobacco, recreational drugs
- Inactivity: being a couch potato, making excuses, procrastinating
- Mental: worrying, obsessing, judging, second guessing, blaming, fussing
- Structurally impaired maxilla with narrow palate

All of these are potential nasal obstructors, particularly if your maxilla is already underdeveloped. Add the following to get snoring: low thyroid, weak adrenals and stomach acid is down from aging and stress, and a standard American diet rich in empty calories and health disruptors.

Before we look into a few cases, it's helpful to know that your nasal passage is a tunnel through your maxilla which comes with air-warming chambers in it called sinuses. The floor of the nose is the roof of the palate, which is why an upper oral appliance can improve breathing by widening the side walls of nasal tunnel in Zones 1 and 2. By contrast, mandibular advancement devices cannot deliver this benefit.

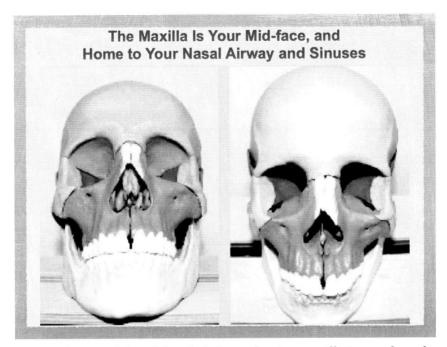

Frontal view of dental-facial skeleton showing maxilla in purple and nasal tunnel through it.

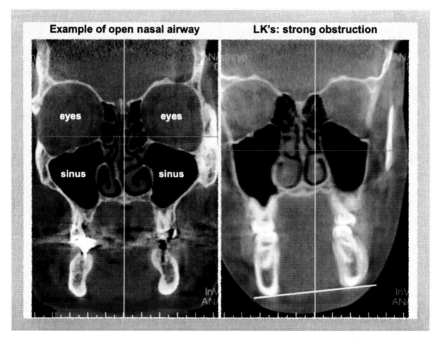

Example of open nasal airway | **LK's: strong obstruction**

In CT images, black is air space while grey is tissue to filter, warm, and humidify incoming air. Left image: Functional nasal passage with open corridors for oxygen delivery suggesting healthy diet. Right image: Strong nasal obstruction from inflammatory diet with slanted lower jaw from Impaired Mouth Syndrome. Yellow line shows an unevenly hinged lower jaw that contributes to neck pain.

A Chairside Chat on Nasal Obstruction

LK, age 19, came with complaints of upper back pain, anxiety, and stress since age 12. Her braces came off at age 11 without extraction of adult teeth. She'd wake up tired about four times a week. Her nasal obstruction is nearly total, as the left image in the slide above shows.

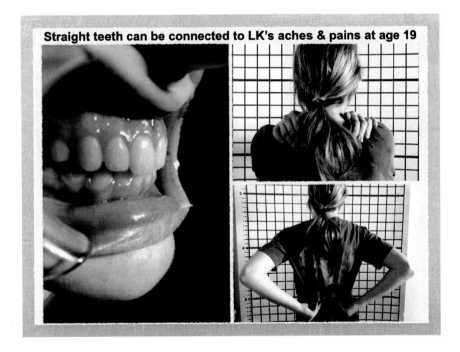

Straight teeth can be connected to LK's aches & pains at age 19

LK had woken with a sinus headache the morning her mom came for her case explanation. "What did she have for dinner last night?" I asked.

"Pasta."

"That makes sense," I replied. "Look at how her airway is closed down on her CT images, especially narrow where the adenoid is enlarged."

"Oh, no!" Mom was instantly alarmed. "She needs her adenoids and tonsils out? I'm not in favor of medication or surgery. What would you do for your own kid?"

"I'd talk to my kid's doctor about this 2010 study[4]. It found better sleep scores after surgical removal of adenoids and tonsils, but only about a quarter of the kids (27.2%) experienced complete resolution of their sleep apnea."

"A 72% failure is not good," she said. "So, what'd you do for your own child?"

"I'd use a WholeHealth approach, which combines oral expander appliance therapy and Buteyko breathing exercises with eating right to reduce nasal swelling. Again, talk with your doctor first."

Mom looked relieved. "How would the appliance help?"

"Widening her palate with an appliance also widens her nasal corridor to improve air flow. The roof of the palate is the floor of the nose."

"I see. But if that works, why does she need to change her way of eating?"

"First, she'll feel better from less nasal congestion. Secondly, she'd look better because mouth-breathing makes a long and narrow horsey face. Lastly, her results will hold better, with less teeth re-crowding."

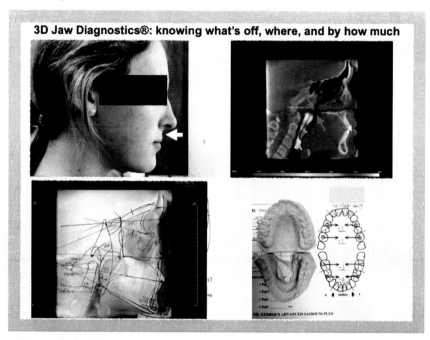

Upper left: White arrow points to Liao's Sign, suggesting a strongly retruded upper jaw. Upper right: Severe upper airway obstruction. The nearly non-existent black space between the two red arrows explains her pain and fatigue; enlarged adenoids further choke her already narrow airway.

Ninety-five percent of my new patients have deficient maxilla based on my 3D Jaw Diagnostics evaluation, and 75% have a stuffy nose, leading to mouth breathing by day and snoring by night. These findings are highly relevant to treatment success.

Redeveloping the "3-foot cage" using both oral appliances and a bone-building diet can help restore healthy nasal function naturally—without surgery, medications, and their side effects. It only takes an inspired patient.

WholeHealth Integration for Upper Airway

Greater nasal volume indeed follows maxilla redevelopment using epigenetic (aka, biomimetic) oral appliances. "Use of these biomimetic appliances might improve continuous positive airway pressure (CPAP) compliance in adults diagnosed with obstructive sleep apnea (OSA), by increasing the nasal cavity volume and decreasing nasal airflow resistance," concludes this 2016 study[5].

With maxillary (upper) epigenetic oral appliances, nasal symptoms improve consistently and predictably. One patient's stuffy nose "went poof" and opened up after 4 weeks. After 9 months, a life-long asthmatic has not had to use her asthma inhaler for over 18 months as of this writing. An initially skeptical surgeon became a believer when he suddenly could breathe through both nostrils after 8 weeks of epigenetic maxillary appliance—this after two sinus surgeries had failed to provide relief.

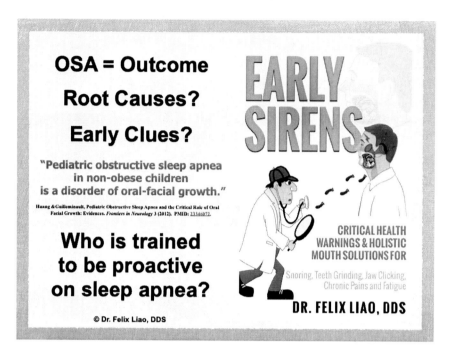

Maxillary appliance can mitigate against colds/flu too, by improving nasal function. After 9 months, Andrea S reported: "In addition to having my neck pain down from 8 on a scale of 10 to 1, I got a significant boost in my immune system." She continued:

> "I have a 7- and 2-year old, so there are always germs around…I'd catch it every time they got it, even if I washed my hands. Usually I'd be down for 2 weeks with significant symptoms. Recently, I got a cold, but it was only 3 days and I only needed an OTC and I was able to go to work. Last year, I was sick every month, and once I vomited at work from a cold, and I was out for a week. No day out of work this year."

A functional upper airway requires a wide-open Zones 1, 2, and 3 from a fully developed maxilla. That's why snoring and mouth-breathers hear from me about food sensitivity first, and bone-building diet second (chapter 23).

Food Sensitivity (or Intolerance) and Nasal Obstruction

Your mouth Style affects your nose and sleep through food sensitivity, aka intolerances. "Over 60% of the population know they must avoid certain foods. Many others are not aware they have food sensitivities. Many think that fatigue, itchy skin or a runny nose are 'normal,'" writes Dr. Lawrence Wilson, MD in his blogpost[6].

Food sensitivity reactions do not involve the immune system, whereas food allergy does. For example, peanut allergy can kill by shutting the throat with swelling (anaphylaxis), whereas food sensitivity does not threaten life. With Dr. Wilson's kind permission, here is his list of food sensitivity causes: digestive and enzyme deficiencies, leaky gut syndrome, food variety and processing, and poor eating habits.

In my view, aging, stress, and lower body temperature are aggravators, but so is Dr. Wilson's point here: "Eating on the run, eating too fast, eating when anxious, eating too much, drinking too much water or other beverages with meals, or eating ice cold or scalding foods can all impair the digestion process." Do you need to reform your mouth Style?

Despite oral appliance therapy, snoring and mouth breathing will persist if habitual mouth Style stays unchanged. Dr. Wilson writes, "… some people can drink natural, whole milk, but not pasteurized, homogenized milk from cows injected with bovine growth hormone and fed antibiotics. Many foods contain pesticide residues, as well as a chemical soup of up to twenty or thirty additives, preservatives, artificial flavors, colors, and other chemicals - all in one food!"

Are you starting to see how LK woke up with a sinus headache at a young age, and why she needs to change her mouth style for full resolution? Her case is typical, not an exception.

Getting Back to Ethnic Roots and Whole Foods: Arun's Case

Arun, age 10, was brought by his dad for crowded teeth, sleep apnea, and habitual mouth breathing, despite having his tonsils and adenoids removed at age 3 after a diagnosis of obstructive sleep apnea. His lips stayed apart during the entire visit. I called it to his dad's attention and said, "If his stuffy nose isn't addressed first, all your investment in his jaw development will likely relapse later."

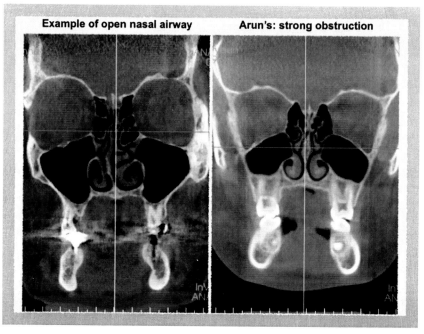

Right: Normal nasal passage and sinus. Left: A case of strong nasal obstruction and sinus congestion in a 9-year-old with habitual mouth breathing.

"So, what can we do?" Dad asked.

"Start giving him your native Indian diet. Stop the standard American diet, which is bad for his airway, as Dr. Wilson explained. Minimize processed foods that come in packages and boxes and give him whole foods from responsible growers and pristine sources as much as you can."

"That's going to be hard—he *loves* pizza!"

"That's why he has Americanized airway and jaw problems. Feed him grandma's cooking, made with TLC. It's how humankind—and your own family—have come this far. To reach his genetic potential while growing up in America, I recommend that you visit Weston A. Price Foundation[7] to learn Nourishing Traditions Diet's principles first. Then explore ethnic foods—Chinese, Italian, Mexican, etc., and your grandma's home cooking."

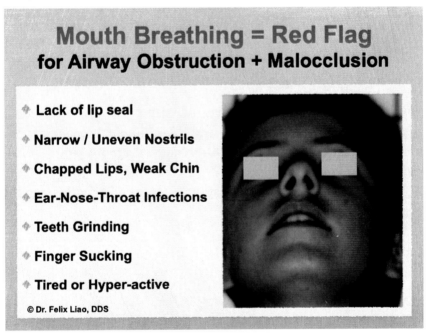

Lip seal is a pre-requisite for optimal dental-facial development because the lips, cheeks, and tongue are more powerful than appliances and braces to shape faces and smiles. That's why fixing impaired mouth Structure starts with eating a non-congestive diet. Non-medication approach to sinusitis[8] is an informative podcast by Dr. Steven Park, MD, who is also the author of *Sleep Interrupted.*

Breathing First, Then Dental Work

Dr. CJ emailed me about a month after she had started AMD training with me. She was concerned that she might be over-diagnosing airway issues. "Over the last several weeks, during my hygiene checkups, it seems that about 8/10 patients have several risk factors that may contribute to sleep/airway disorder. I am seeing so much more than before. It's kinda scary."

"Eight of ten parallels my experience," I assured her. "Congratulations—you've grown new eyes. Screening is not yet diagnosis. The next two steps are (1) a sleep test for medical diagnosis, and (2) airway records to establish what's off, where, and by how much to design your oral appliances."

Dr. CJ continued: "I am attaching my daughter's CT scan image because she grinds very loudly and very anxiously at night. She also tosses and turns in her sleep, and in the morning, I can tell she didn't have a good night's sleep. I can't wait to treat her with your guidance...Thank you for opening my eyes to this and helping me treat my patients."

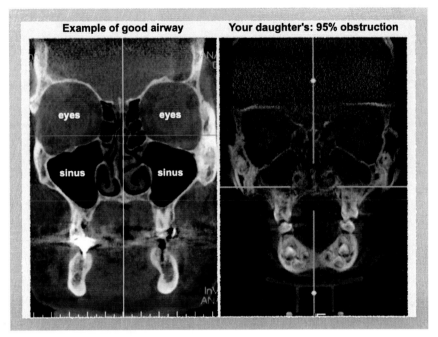

A case of nearly total nasal obstruction and sinus congestion in a 9-year-old. In the right image, there's almost no black in sinus spaces, nor in the nasal passage, meaning near-total obstruction of nasal airway and sinuses—and thus full-time mouth breathing detrimental to optimal dental-facial development.

Finally, "Pregnant women—especially those with allergies— should be aware that their diet during pregnancy can affect their child's chances of developing eczema and/or food allergies," noted Dr. David Fleischer MD, co-author of a 2019 study reported by Medscape[9]. "Vaginal delivery and breast-feeding diminish the incidence of allergy and asthma in children up to the age of 18."

You cannot control your gestation or upbringing, but you can adopt a holistic mouth Style to eat smarter and fix stuffy nose and snoring at the source.

WholeHealth Integration

- Fixing impaired mouth Structure starts with eating a non-congestive diet. An appliance by itself does not heal the patient. It takes a doctor with knowledge, experience, a healer's heart, and WholeHealth team of experts.

- Patients: Find an AMD (Airway-centered Mouth Doctor®) to help get your stuffy nose resolved in combination with oral appliances and fully open your airway to support deep sleep.

- AMDs: Read up on food sensitivity and find a functional medicine expert in your community to work with to get all patients—young and old—back on the right track.

- Dentists: Consider taking AMD Training to grow new eyes and start making a bigger difference for your patients with root-cause diagnoses, treatment, and referrals.

- Non-dentist HCPs: Reach out to AMDs in your community and start collaborating on gut health restoration and sleep support through nasal and pharyngeal airway redevelopment using epigenetic oral appliances.

Chapter 19

'Pleasantly Surprised': Erectile Dysfunction Gone and CPAP Mask Bye-bye

"Health is a state of complete physical, mental and social well-being and not merely the absence of disease or infirmity."

~ World Health Organization[1]

The benefits of nasal breathing are many: fewer colds or bouts of flu, better-tasting food, less anxiety, improved circulation, better sex, and more. That's because nasal breathing makes nitric oxide (NO), the magic ingredient for cardiovascular health and erectile dysfunction.

Nitric oxide "is one of the most important molecules produced in the human body," says leading expert Dr. Nathan Bryan[2]. "It regulates many important cell functions including regulation of healthy blood flow and healthy blood pressure levels, communication between cells in the brain as well as how our body defends itself against pathogens."

"Nasal NO may have important local as well as distal effects in, for example, host defense and regulation of pulmonary function," concludes this 1999 British Medical Journal Review[3].

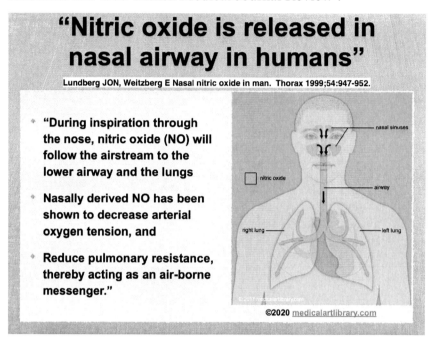

"Nitric oxide is released in nasal airway in humans"

Lundberg JON, Weitzberg E Nasal nitric oxide in man. Thorax 1999;54:947-952.

* "During inspiration through the nose, nitric oxide (NO) will follow the airstream to the lower airway and the lungs

* Nasally derived NO has been shown to decrease arterial oxygen tension, and

* Reduce pulmonary resistance, thereby acting as an air-borne messenger."

nasal sinuses

nitric oxide

airway

right lung

left lung

©2020 medicalartlibrary.com

Nasal Breathing Supports Immunity

Nitric oxide can block the viral replication cycle of severe acute respiratory syndrome coronavirus (SARS CoV), according to this 2005 Swedish study[4]. "We also show here that NO inhibits viral protein and RNA synthesis."

Translated: NO from nose-breathing can mitigate respiratory infections. "Nasally derived NO has been shown to increase arterial oxygen tension and reduce pulmonary vascular resistance, thereby acting as an airborne messenger," confirmed another 1999 study in *Thorax*[5].

Wonderful as it is, you can't just go out and buy nitric oxide, because it's an unstable gas made inside your body. Dr. Bryan notes two pathways for NO production[6]: (1) through an enzyme inside your blood vessel lining and (2) a diet rich in dark, leafy greens such as spinach, kale, and beets." These vegetables are rich in nitrates, but their conversion to nitric oxide can be blocked by poor oral hygiene, mouthwash overuse, and oral infections.

NO in turn is oxygen-driven: "Oxygen plays a predominant role in Nitric Oxide (NO) activity," emphasizes a 2015 overview article[7]. Epigenetic oral appliances can widen airway, which then means more oxygen and nitric oxide—which, in turn, means healthy vascular function.

'Pleasantly Surprised': Fred's Case

Fred was a career military officer whose presenting complaints included brain fog ("I just can't get things done"); waking up tired despite BIPAP (a newer version of CPAP); very dry mouth in the morning; increased daytime sleepiness; erectile dysfunction; aches and pains in his hamstrings, Achilles, and the right side of his neck; and TMJ dysfunction.

Fred wanted to treat the real root cause. He didn't want to have to rely on a machine forever to sleep. Fred had tried BIPAP four months before turning to me for epigenetic oral appliance therapy. "Prior to the sleep test diagnosis," he said, "I used to wake up violently after not being able to breathe about three hours later. Without BIPAP, it'd mess me up the next day."

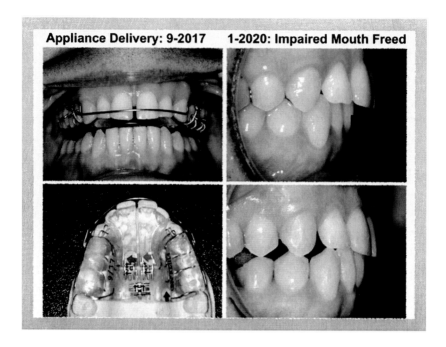

And after he began wearing his appliances 14 hours a day? "I went off CPAP on my own and my energy feels the same as with CPAP." Just read his testimony:

> "It's now almost two years since I started the DNA appliance…One day I fell asleep without CPAP and without appliance, and I woke up feeling just fine, which is totally unlike before. So I stopped CPAP a month ago and used just the appliance when I sleep. My energy feels the same as with CPAP, except not lugging equipment when I travel."

It had an effect on his erectile dysfunction, too:

> "At around 11 months after starting oral appliances, I'd wake up a lot at night with nocturnal erections, which was something that…rarely if ever happened before I started using the device. But it happens frequently now and sometimes multiple times a night…I am pleasantly surprised. I wonder if they are advertising the wrong thing at football games."

As always, patient compliance is key to treatment success, along with doctor diagnosis and appliance design. One case does not make a pattern, but we can see Fred's result as another confirmation that adults' jaws *can* be redeveloped epigenetically to widen the airway and thereby restore heart, brain, and also sexual function.

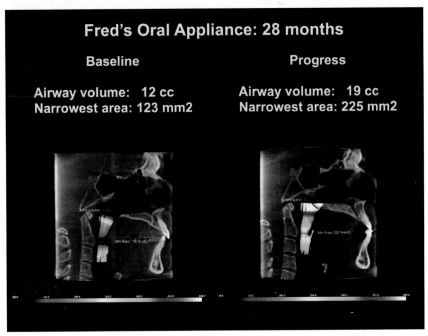

Fred's Oral Appliance: 28 months

Baseline

Airway volume: 12 cc
Narrowest area: 123 mm2

Progress

Airway volume: 19 cc
Narrowest area: 225 mm2

Erectile dysfunction gone with bigger airway volume by 58% and narrowest cross section wider by 83% from epigenetic oral appliance and 100% patient compliance in this case.

Erectile Dysfunction: A Canary for Circulation and Airway

Erectile dysfunction is a red flag for cardiovascular decline and systemic damage. As with most degenerative diseases, many factors and multiple systems are involved in ED. "Sleep fragmentation and, to a lesser extent, hypoxia in addition to the degree of obesity and aging may be responsible for the central suppression of testosterone in these patients," found this 2002 study[8].

Nitric oxide is also made in the inner lining (endothelium) of your blood vessels to signal surrounding muscles to relax. This increases blood flow and lowers blood pressure. "Loss of NO function is one of the earliest indicators or markers of disease," states a study in 2011 Journal of Geriatric Cardiology[9]. The study also states:

> "Clinical studies provide evidence that insufficient NO production is associated with all major cardiovascular risk factors, such as hyperlipidemia, diabetes, hypertension, smoking and severity of atherosclerosis, and also has a profound predictive value for disease progression including cardiovascular and Alzheimer's disease."

Nitric oxide goes down with age. It's the difference between vigorous youth and grumpy old men. A poor lifestyle can mean a 90% NO decline by age 50 per the study above, compared to just a 20% decline with a healthy lifestyle. You are not only what you eat, but also how you sleep, breathe, work, play, and how you eat.

Taking a pill advertised on TV for "Low-T" may mask a symptom and miss a serious root cause. "Recognizing ED as a disease marker for CVD [cardio-vascular disease] may help to identify individuals at risk for having a premature cardiovascular event," finds a 2011 Cardiology Review[10].

Heart disease can kill, often without much lead time. Sudden cardiac death is not a heart attack, but an abrupt malfunction in the heart's electrical system that disrupts blood supply to the brain. "Sudden cardiac death [SCD] is the largest single cause of natural death in the United States…SCD is responsible for half of heart disease deaths," according to Cleveland Clinic[11]. "In over half of the cases, however, sudden cardiac arrest occurs without prior symptoms."

Can erectile dysfunction be an early clue? "Most cases of erectile dysfunction (ED) recognize a vascular etiology," states a 2003 editorial in European Urology[12]. "Common risk factors for atherosclerosis have been frequently found in patients with ED. ED may be considered as the clinical manifestation of a disease affecting penile circulation as a part of a more generalized vascular disorder."

Circulation feeds the entire body, including each and every tooth. If oxygen and nitric oxide can relax the penile artery, the same can happen to the oxygen-starved tissues inside a screaming achy tooth, if the circulation is restored within 24 to 36 hours from the very first pain—see chapter 11 in *Early Sirens*. Conversely, the longer you let Impaired Mouth Syndrome and sleep apnea slide, the more likely your teeth will suffer root canal "nerve death" from oxygen deprivation.

Finally, circulation carries more than oxygen. It also brings what typical Americans eat—a crazy excess of added sugar, fats, salt, plastics, herbicides, and environmental toxins—to degenerate dental nerves and clog the penile artery.

Liquid Oxygen Supplementation

On a Sunday morning when I could sleep to my heart's content, I took my blood pressure on waking up and then every 15 minutes after sniffing half a dropper of a proprietary liquid oxygen supplement in saline into each nostril. Sniffing bypasses the gut and takes the oxygen directly into the brain, allowing a tiny amount of the supplement to have a sizable effect. It's normal for the upper number to go up as the morning unfolds.

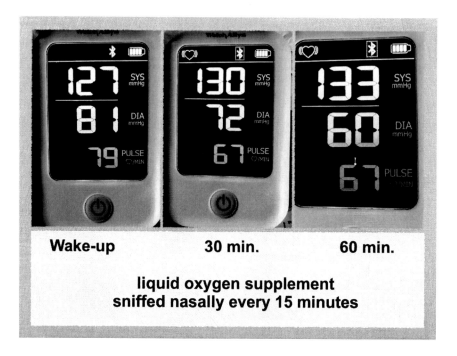

Wake-up   **30 min.**   **60 min.**

**liquid oxygen supplement
sniffed nasally every 15 minutes**

Noteworthy is how my resting blood pressure dropped 25% (from 81 to 60) with the oxygen supplement, and my heart rate (HR) dropped 15%. "HR not only reflects the status of the cardiovascular system," states a 2014 study[13] in circulation, "but also serves as an indicator of cardiac autonomic nervous system activity and metabolic rate."

One case doesn't make a pattern, but my data shows evidence of circulatory relaxation and points to the potential of oxygen supplement to amplify oral appliance therapy and support whole-body health. I also use this liquid oxygen supplement to:

- Unblock nasal obstruction at bedtime in conjunction with Buteyko breathing exercise #114 to alleviate snoring.
- Soothe tired/dry eyes from contact lenses or staring at screens too much.

"I always start with a couple of drops in my dry itchy eyes first thing in the morning," an AMD emailed me. "Not only do the drops soothe my eyes, but I feel refreshed so I don't so much need my coffee as just enjoy it." Indeed, this liquid oxygen supplement supported my eyes and my brain through the research and writing of this book.

With oxygen comes nitric oxide, better cardiovascular health, and higher life quality. Ask your healthcare professionals and AMD how they can help boost your oxygen naturally, painlessly and sustainably.

WholeHealth Integration

- Give your body what it needs, and it will thrive. In nearly every case, it's oxygen first and foremost. With oxygen comes nitric oxide, cardiovascular health, and higher life quality.

- With oxygen and nasal breathing comes nitric oxide, helping you thrive physically, energetically, and sexually—no pills needed. Just adopt a Holistic Mouth Style and redevelop your deficient maxilla.

- Erectile dysfunction is not just about testosterone. It's a local symptom of a more systemic circulatory decline.

- Erectile dysfunction has oral contributions from stress, sleep deprivation, impaired mouth Structure (oxygen deficiency from airway obstruction), and impaired mouth Style of eating a typical American diet steadily leading to atherosclerosis and diabetes.

Chapter 20

Yin and Yang Balance: Your Ticket to Thrive

"Good sleep, good food and exercise are the 3-legged stool that holds up your health. But if I were forced to choose one, it would 100% be good sleep."

~ Cecilia Wu, M.D.,
Anatomic, Forensic and Cardiovascular Pathologist

Baby Boomers are retiring, and heart disease and cancer are still America's leading killers. What's missing? Meantime, rates of costly new illnesses such as sleep apnea and Alzheimer's are rising fast. What happened? More importantly, what can you do proactively to live a full life and depart without agony?

The human body is designed to be self-renewing until your genetic clock runs out. As you've been seeing, sleeping with impaired mouth Structure and eating foods laced with health disruptors can short-change your internal fitness and hasten your "sunset." Carcinogens

241

and radiation can cause cancer. Stress can trigger overeating. The standard American diet, super-processed and high in sugar, brings on obesity and inflammation.

The better you manage those health disruptors, the better your Alignment, Breathing, Circulation, and Digestion systems can work as semi-perpetual energy generators. Let's turn next to a concept from Traditional Chinese Medicine that runs through health and life—Yin/Yang balance—and tie it back to circadian rhythm and Western medicine.

Yin and Yang: An Over-Simplified Overview

Traditional Chinese Medicine (TCM) evolved from farmers' observation of cyclic changes in heaven and on earth. Seasons change and spring returns; light fades as the day wanes and darkness gains. The maximal light at noon is designated as Yang. The shadow then lengthens toward Yin and reaches maximal darkness before light takes over again. This is how days and seasons extend into years, eons, infinity, and how Nature or Cosmos works.

The foundational concept is that Yang is built into Yin, and Yin is built into Yang, as shown in the familiar Tai Chi symbol. *Chi (Qi)* is the Chinese term for the energy that gives rise to life, wellness, and longevity. *Chi* is what holds your joints and body together. Your health falls apart when *Chi* is gone.

In TCM, humans stand between Heaven and Earth, which means the human body is thus subject to the same Yin/Yang cycling in Nature. *Chi* moves the pendulum from Yang to Yin and Yin to Yang. Balance comes from returning to the middle over and over.

Think of Yang as an "on" switch and Yin as "off." What happens if a car comes without a brake? So, balance is important to safety and health. What happens if a mouth comes with an unreliable "off" switch?

Yang uses energy; Yin restores it. What do you think happens to your health and longevity when it's all Yang all the time? That's the case with burning the candle from both ends for years.

Yin-Yang has a parallel in Western medicine: the autonomic nervous system (ANS) in charge of your survival and renewal. ANS is classically divided into:

- The Sympathetic nervous system (SNS), which activates the fight-or-flight response in the face of stress and threats.
- The Parasympathetic nervous system (PNS), which activates the rest and relaxation response to repair wear and tear.

Here's how Yin-Yang applies illness and wellness:

- Sympathetics Nervous System (SNS) responds to stress with energy expenditure.
- Para-Sympathetics (PNS) restores daily wear and tear.
- Balancing SNS/PNS equals sustainable health and wellness.
- Chronic stress blocks PNS healing and perpetuates inflammation.
- Depleted SNS: gets sick easily and delays recovery.

Optimal health (with the slowest decline) is sustainable when Sympathetics (Yang) are on during the day and Parasympathetics (Yin) are on during the hours of darkness. This way, the body stays in the zone of balance (self-regulation).

When Yin-Yang are out of balance, health goes downhill faster and comes back slower—sound familiar?

Sleep = Down Time, or Active Time?

- Kids' growth and adults' repairs requires deep sleep
- Renew daytime neurotransmitters: histamine (awake), dopamine (get done), serotonin (feel good)
- Consolidate learning + memory
- Process daily waste for release in AM
- Empowers Immunity + heals Illness
- Deficient oxygen = impaired health
- Weight loss = diet + exercise + sleep

© Dr. Felix Liao, DDS

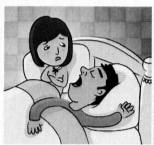

Sympathetic Dominance: When Do You Rest?

A visiting professor from Poland once came to see me for a dental emergency. Afterward, I asked for his impression of America and he chuckled. "We work five and a half days in Poland, then we rest," he said. "You Americans work hard five days and play harder on weekends. So, when do you rest?!"

Stress is stress, whether it's physical (freezing cold outside, say, or hypothyroid inside), mental (for instance, a broken record in your head repeating, "You are never good enough"), or emotional (blindsided by layoff, betrayal, sudden death, etc.), or a lifestyle of all work and party with no rest. Your stress response is either on or off, just like your smartphone.

Your ANS perceives only "threat" or "no threat," activation or stand down, fight or relax. Responding to an alarm clock and checking all the boxes day after day is like stepping on the gas pedal to activate your Sympathetic's Yang. Initially, your body responds quickly and smoothly, and you enjoy revving it up. Prolonged peak performance and a jam-packed schedule over time results in wear and tear. Staying in the overheated red zone over time can tip your body into sympathetic dominance. The following diagram is worth another look from this perspective.

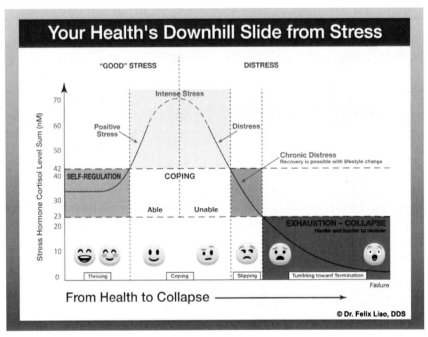

Sympathetic dominance on the downslope (right half of the yellow box) means distress—your "tail is pinched" by a clamp beyond your reach for too long, and your ability to cope is fading. Recall that eating is a dominant stress response that can override your "I know better" rational brain. Indulging your sweet tooth becomes an escape at a price of inflammation. So is relying on caffeinated or "energy" drinks, munching, and drinking. For evidence of tampered-with, hyper-processed foods you've consumed, look at the packages in your trash can.

Sympathetic dominance combines with impaired mouth Style to promote obesity, heart disease, autoimmune disorders, and susceptibility to infections.

When your body's "Go" switch is perpetually on and wired to "high," your energy will end up depleted, with less in the tank for comeback (the orange box in the image above) in the fight against cancer or infections. The death spiral comes when either Yin or Yang are simply too weak for a comeback. Recovery from the red zone is longer and costlier, if at all.

It takes energy to come back up the hill. How can you do that with an empty tank?

Staying well and recovering lost health follows the same rule: dial down Sympathetic dominance. The difference is WHEN — after you fall ill, or before—in a hospital, or in your own home.

Restoring Yin is a simple and effective remedy for reversing chronic illness and avoiding premature aging. You can rebalance Yin/Yang with the Proactive Wellness Care (chapter 15), restore deep sleep by widening obstructed airway, and douse inflammation with a healthier mouth Style.

Just as "go west" was the advice that developed 19th century America, "go Yin" is the prescription that most of us 21st century Americans would do well to take. The Vagus Nerve is how you go Yin.

The Vagus Nerve: Power Cord to Your Gut-Brain Axis

Eating involves tasting and chewing and secreting saliva, which are just some functions of the Vagus Nerve (VN). VN is the Yin (restorative) half of your autonomic nervous system.

"Vagus" is the Latin word for wandering, which describes this nerve perfectly. VN is the longest and most complex of the twelve cranial nerves, starting inside your brain case and running through your chest and gut, ending in the pelvic floor. VN powers all your internal organs from the throat down and connects them with your brain. VN feeds gut conditions to the brain to maintain self-regulation, which in turn regulates digestion and inflammation. VN is the data cable powering the gut-brain axis both ways.

The key functions VN regulates include digestion, heartbeat, blinking, breathing depth and speed, opening and closing of blood vessels and sweat glands, detoxification via the liver and kidneys, bowel movement, urination, and sexual arousal.

Your VN is also for social engagement that promotes survival. The emotions on your face (facial affect) is revealed by VN. Depression comes with a flat facial affect, and motherly love is unmistakably clear. We humans are endowed with an instinctive ability to read a face to ensure survival.

VN helps us make split-second decisions on friend or foe, which can mean luck or disaster, or even life or death. Non-mammals don't have this ability. A cold-blooded lizard, when faced with a threat, has just two options: flee or freeze (play dead). The former spends energy (go Yang); the latter saves it (go Yin).

The more evolved VN in humans and other mammals comes with multiple cables—as Dr. Stephen Porges explains in his Polyvagal Theory[1]:

"The 'newer' myelinated ventral vagal motor pathways regulate supra-diaphragmatic organs (e.g., heart and lungs) and are integrated in the brain stem with structures that regulate the striated muscles of the face and head...resulting in a functional social engagement system."

Your VN participates in your social and relational well-being by connecting facial affect with the gut-brain axis. Poly-vagal theory has catalyzed a whole new field of research on the treatment of trauma with safety at its core.

You can see PNS on the face of someone asleep: peaceful, almost angelic. In the Yang/Sympathetic dominance mode, we are human doings. In the Yin/PNS mode, we are human beings.

Strong Vagus Tone: Your Ticket to Thrive

Inflammation is a normal response to infections, bodily injuries, and stress. When your body can self-regulate well, inflammation initiates healing and is self-limiting. That requires a high-functioning strong Vagus Nerve (VN).

When your VN is dysfunctional—made worse with thyroid insufficiency and adrenal depletion—inflammation can turn chronic and initiate degenerative and killer diseases:

- Alzheimer's in the brain.
- Arthritis in the joints.
- Asthma in the chest.
- Ulcerative colitis and Crohn's in the gut.
- High blood pressure and atherosclerosis in circulation system.
- Diabesity (diabetes plus obesity).
- Autoimmune diseases or cancer anywhere.

One sign of a strong VN is a lower heart rate. For instance, a 1997 study[2] in the *Journal of the American College of Cardiologists* noted that, "Among mammals, there is an inverse semilogarithmic relation between heart rate and life expectancy." Translated: Lower heart rate means greater longevity.

Conversely, a 2019 Swedish Study[3] found that "high RHR [resting heart rate 75 beats per minute or higher] was associated with an increased risk of death and cardiovascular events in men from the general population." Higher heart rate means your heart is working harder, and overdrive cannot outlast low and steady.

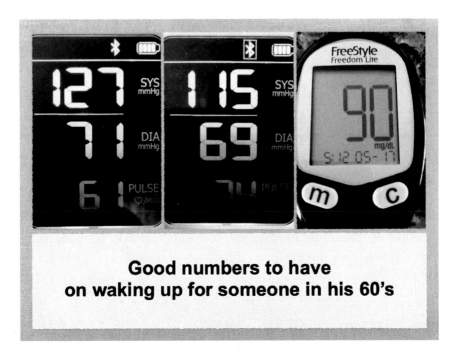

**Good numbers to have
on waking up for someone in his 60's**

A strong vagus is your "ticket to thrive." A weak vagus starts many health problems, says Dr. Navaz Habib in *Activate Your Vagus Nerve*[4]. Here's my super-condensed summary with his generous permission:

- Obstructive Sleep Apnea: Airway collapse can come from flaccid pharyngeal [throat] muscles.
- Heart Rate: VN "has a major role in ensuring that the heart rate stays within a comfortable range when the body is not under stress."
- Blood Pressure: VN "relays information to and from the kidneys...thus managing the overall blood pressure of the body."
- Overeating: "In order to be satiated, we require signals from the liver.... An under-active VN may not be able to effectively send this signal."
- High Blood Sugar: "The inability to shift back [from stress to recovery mode] leads the liver to continuously produce glucose, leading to higher blood sugar level in the longer term."

- Dinner Size and Time: "The sensitivity of the stomach [regulated by VN] decreases at night, so we are more likely to overeat later in the evening."
- Pain from Bile Stagnation, Chronic Constipation, and Diarrhea.
- Gut Inflammation: "Much research shows that activation of the VN actually reduces the inflammation…"
- Chest Breathing: "The first and most common cause of dysfunctional signaling in VN is dysfunctional breathing."

Your fight/flight sympathetic system lives in your chest, while your restorative parasympathetic system resides mainly in your belly. You can check yourself by putting one hand on your chest and the other over your navel and inhale. Does your upper hand go up? If yes, you're likely a chest breather with a weaker vagus.

You need a strong VN to restore Yin and to thrive. Breathing lessons are beyond the scope of this book, but they are part of the Smart Health Keeping™ webinars—see Resources. Next, let's go to the best part: eating.

WholeHealth Integration

- Learning to restore Yin-Yang balance early on is a critical personal wellness skill, just like toothbrushing and knowing how to eat.

- Impaired Mouth Structure + Style = miserable life with adrenal exhaustion, no joy, premature aging, earlier death with big medical bills.

- The same rule applies to staying well and recovering lost health: dial down Sympathetic dominance (Yang excess). The difference is whether you "go Yin" to regain balance in time, or too late.

- A strong Vagus Nerve is your "ticket to thrive," while a weak Vagus Nerve starts chronic inflammation and degenerative killer diseases.

Chapter 21

Getting Your License to Thrive

Fear less, hope more; Eat less, chew more;
Whine less, breathe more; Talk less, say more;
Hate less, love more; And all
good things are yours.

~ Swedish Proverb

Thriving health starts with restorative sleep and nourishing nutrients for your body to run its own house. Many Americans suffer from both impaired mouth Structure and Stye. The next 2 slides show four of them who grew up eating standard American diet, getting medical and dental checkups, and exercising regularly.

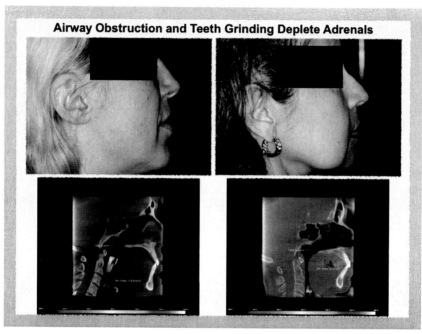

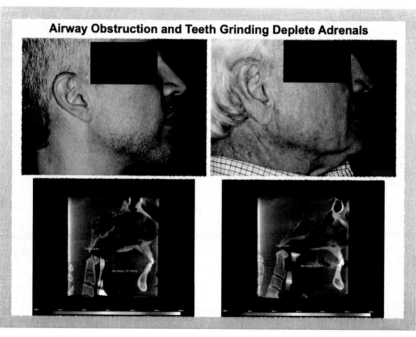

What do they need to start feeling great, looking vibrant—naturally and sustainably, starting now—and aging well going forward?

Thriving means having all the energy your body needs to support health, resist disease, heal faster, and stand up to gravity's perpetual pull toward the grave. It translates into spring in your step, gas in your tank, sunshine in your heart, and glow on your face. That energy to thrive comes through your mouth from daily food and nightly sleep.

Holistic Mouth Solutions cover both Structure and Style. The prior chapters give you the science. This chapter starts getting you licensed to thrive by developing your Holistic Mouth Style as an essential wellness skill to keep your waist lean, gut clean, inflammation low, and immunity up.

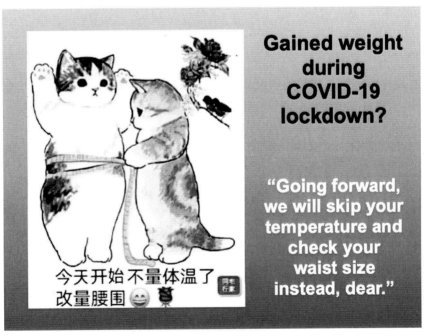

Seventy-six percent of medical doctors admit to gaining weight during COVID-19 pandemic lockdown in Medscape's survey in May 2020[1].

Thriver's Training

Thriver's training helps you acquire Holistic Mouth Style and grow it into a healthful habit like toothbrushing and doing yoga. It turns you from a susceptible consumer into a confident owner-operator of your mouth. Instead of feeding your body with pre-made foods in packages, you will learn to nourish yourself by knowing how to make tasty and healthy food in your own kitchen.

Thriving health is both our destination and journey. Reducing inflammation and enhancing renewal naturally through food and sleep is our main focus. Thriver's training is about shedding your sweet tooth rather than forbidding sweets. Weight loss is not the primary goal, although it's frequently a positive side effect of turning Holistic Mouth Style into a wellness habit.

Mouth Structure and Style as Root Causes of Health Troubles

Why do modern American patients come to me with a mask of pain and fatigue on their worried and suffering faces, and bunched up teeth and narrow palate in their mouths? How do I get my patients to go in the right direction again?

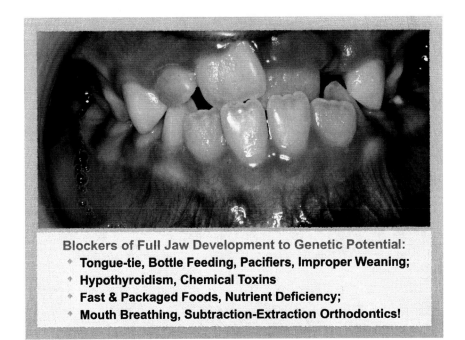

Blockers of Full Jaw Development to Genetic Potential:
- Tongue-tie, Bottle Feeding, Pacifiers, Improper Weaning;
- Hypothyroidism, Chemical Toxins
- Fast & Packaged Foods, Nutrient Deficiency;
- Mouth Breathing, Subtraction-Extraction Orthodontics!

Dr. Weston A. Price's *Nutrition and Physical Degeneration*[2] offers the answer. He had traveled the world and found natives in different parts of the world with fully developed dental arches, naturally straight teeth, radiant faces, and joyous disposition.

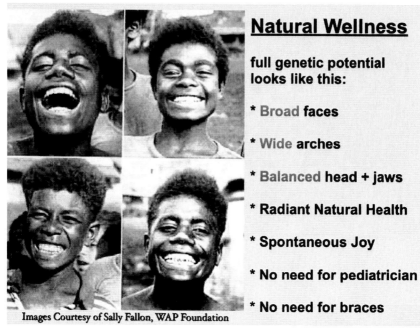

Natural Wellness

full genetic potential
looks like this:

* Broad faces

* Wide arches

* Balanced head + jaws

* Radiant Natural Health

* Spontaneous Joy

* No need for pediatrician

* No need for braces

Images Courtesy of Sally Fallon, WAP Foundation

Dr. Weston A. Price's natives with fully developed dental-facial skeleton.

Dr. Price's natives are joined by their Taiwan counterparts pictured next. I had visited their new restaurant featuring their native dishes. They had never seen a dentist or pediatrician, nor a gym—just like our ancestors.

What do those natives have that we modern first world people don't?

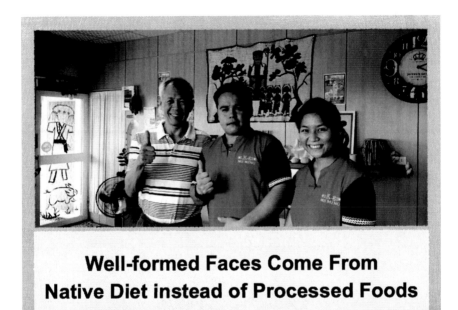

Well-formed Faces Come From Native Diet instead of Processed Foods

Taiwan aborigines (in red tops) with dental-facial features similar to Dr. Price's natives.

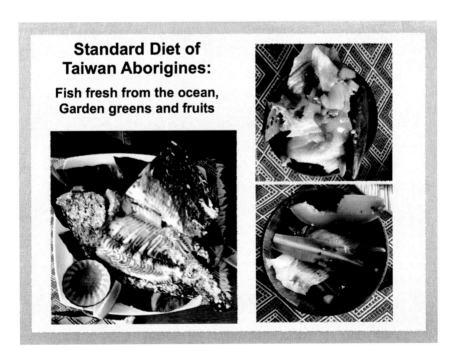

Standard Diet of Taiwan Aborigines:

Fish fresh from the ocean, Garden greens and fruits

Answer: fully developed jaws with room for all teeth. It's not the skin color or geographic origin. Good-looking faces with natural radiance come from wide airway that follows jaw development to full genetic potential. Add fresh whole foods and you just might come close to your genetic potential.

Whether you are ethnically white, black, brown, or mixed, you will suffer medical, dental, mood, and sleep problems if you are stuck with deficient jaws and Impaired Mouth Syndrome.

In my observation, the longer a family tree has been in a westernized society with its white flour, packaged and fast foods, and 24x7 indoor lifestyle with year-round air conditioning, the worse the jaw under-development in each successive generation.

The great news: deficient jaws can be redeveloped regardless of your heritage or age. Impaired Mouth Syndrome can be treated with Holistic Mouth Solutions.

Holistic Mouth Solutions Start Here

The fully-formed jaws and faces of Dr. Price's and my Taiwan natives have inspired me to see a new solution for those suffering Impaired Mouth Syndrome: combining modern epigenetic oral appliances with traditional whole foods made fresh in your own kitchen—just like grandma's old-world cooking.

The magic is not in the mouthpiece, nor in eating a perfect diet, but in their combination to bring out your full genetic potential. All you need is enough healthy natural teeth and a willingness to make the necessary changes. Subtraction orthodontic cases do require more time, cost, and patience.

Focusing on nutrition without ruling out airway obstruction ("3-foot cage") gets you partway there. The same with redeveloping jaws without providing bone-building ingredients. Attending to both mouth Structure and Style can bring breakthrough success.

Chapter 22

Holistic Mouth Style Upgrades Health and Energy

"One of the most important factors in your health will be your ability to bring yourself back to a parasympathetic [recovering] state from a sympathetic [stressed] state. Patients that tend to get better faster and experience amazing results are the ones that learn to create positive lifestyle habits."

~ Dr. Navaz Habib,
Activate Your Vagus Nerve[1]

Your mouth Style is how you use your mouth to eat, drink, and relate to people and Planet Earth, as mentioned. Holistic Mouth Style integrates all three parts of your brain (primitive, emotional, and cognitive) to turn mindless eating into mindful nourishing.

The daily hustle of getting your to-do list completed is a Yang mode activating your "fight or flight" response. Eating and sleeping requires a Yin mode to digest and renew. Knowing how to restore that Yin-Yang balance is essential to helping your health thrive.

How much of your 24-hour day do you spend in Yin versus Yang? As owner of your body and operator of your mouth, you have plenty of control to adopt these positive habits:

- Implementing sleep hygiene to initiate relaxation and sleep
- Monitoring your blood sugar and blood pressure at home
- Cutting down your time spent sitting
- Keeping your mental desktop in peaceful order
- Adding variety, balance, and kindness to your eating habits

Let's take a brief look at each of them.

About Sleep Hygiene

Sleep hygiene is how well your bedroom and bedtime routine promote good sleep. This is especially crucial for people with OSA and obesity because they are oxygen-deprived, adrenally depleted, and Vagus-compromised already.

Good sleep hygiene starts with a pre-requisite: a wide-open airway! If you have a "tiger" tongue inside your mouth, see a qualified AMD or risk getting only limited value from implementing sleep hygiene.

Tongue Crenation = OSA Risk (Teeth Prints on Sides of Tongue)

- 71% specific for sleep efficiency < 85%.
- 70% specific for OSA: AHI > 5
- 86% specific for oxygen concentration drop ≥ 4%.
- Weiss et al, The Association of Tongue Scalloping with Obstructive Sleep Apnea and Related Sleep Pathology, 2005. PMID: 16360522
- Note crowded lower front teeth implicating Impaired Mouth Syndrome

© Dr. Felix Liao, DDS

Crenation means less real sleep, higher risk of sleep apnea, and more oxygen deficiency. Crowded lower front teeth means a narrower "cage" for the "tiger" tongue.

Treat your sleep hours like work hours—as if you'll be paid for time asleep. You'll get that "good to go" feeling when you wake up in the morning. The growth hormones for repairing daily wear and tear are released during Yin hours of darkness.

The relaxed Yin state of rest, quiet, and warmth is necessary for your body to make melanin (which gives color to your hair), and then melatonin (the sleep hormone and a powerful brain antioxidant), and finally thyroxine, the precursor of thyroid hormone—great payoff from observing the Chinese Body Clock.

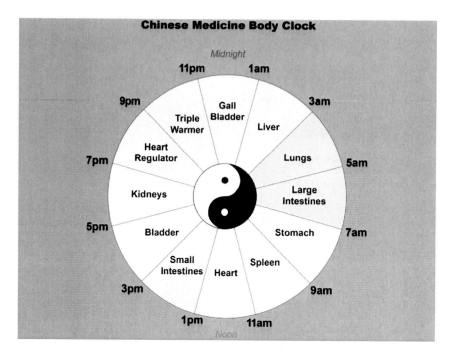

Conversely, when you stay up late night after night for years, you can get these instead: droopy eyelids, hair gone white, thin, and/or bald, body gone fat and cold, erection gone south, and memory going blank.

With his generous permission, the following list of good sleep hygiene tips are adapted from Dr. Jacob Teitelbaum's *From Fatigue to Fantastic!*[2] They cost next to nothing to implement.

- Keep a regular bedtime. Start your shutdown by 10 p.m. so you can be asleep by 11 p.m. to allow 7 to 9 hours of sleep.
- Ban TV and smartphones from your bedroom. Blue light activates stress hormones. Keep your bedroom as a sanctuary for sleep and love only.
- Invest in blackout blinds so you can't see your fingers with your arm extended. No darkness means no growth hormone nor repair. That $80 for a blackout blind over my bedroom window ranks among the smartest money I have ever spent on my health.

- Wind down with sunset. Don't exercise within four hours of bedtime and avoid caffeine after 2 p.m. to avoid disrupting your body clock.
- For dinner, allow 4 hours before bedtime to reduce gut inflammation. If not, have soup and cooked vegetables only. Avoid greasy meats, heavy dairy, and desserts.
- Avoid alcohol after dinner, especially if you are on medications or have a pot belly, sleep apnea, or all the above. Alcohol is a respiratory depressant.
- Monitor your own snoring and breathing with smart devices or have your sleep partner observe your snoring intensity and gasping. A sleep test is best to rule out sleep apnea.

From Fatigues to Fantastic also includes tips on racing minds, snoring sleep partners, bladder wake-ups during sleep, and more.

Monitor Your Blood Sugar and Blood Pressure at Home

Another habit you have full control over is to track your blood sugar and blood pressure. Simply paying attention can help them get better.

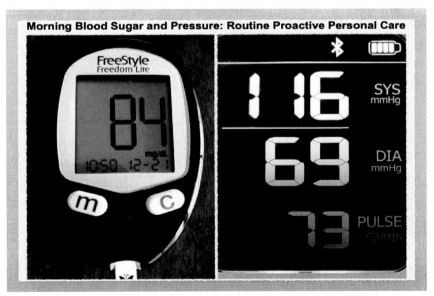

My personal goal is 100 mg/dl. Above 90 is "blinking yellow light." Consult your healthcare professional for your own case.

You can keep diabetes at bay if you stay below pre-diabetic threshold. You can adjust other habits as needed once you can see how your numbers are trending. Ask your doctor for guidance and monitoring.

Healthy & Unhealthy Blood Pressure Ranges
American Heart Association

BLOOD PRESSURE CATEGORY	SYSTOLIC mm Hg (upper number)		DIASTOLIC mm Hg (lower number)
NORMAL	LESS THAN 120	and	LESS THAN 80
ELEVATED	120 – 129	and	LESS THAN 80
HIGH BLOOD PRESSURE (HYPERTENSION) STAGE 1	130 – 139	or	80 – 89
HIGH BLOOD PRESSURE (HYPERTENSION) STAGE 2	140 OR HIGHER	or	90 OR HIGHER
HYPERTENSIVE CRISIS (consult your doctor immediately)	HIGHER THAN 180	and/or	HIGHER THAN 120

Whatever you measure will get better from your attention, be it blood pressure, blood sugar, weight, or hours spent sitting. Wherever your attention is missing, that's when your health slips away. This applies to mental stress too.

Your Mental Desktop

Your mind can be a health asset or a liability. Your attitude affects more than just your stress eating. It affects your customer relationships and friendships too. Do you wear smiles in your mind, or frowns?

Your mood is your quality of life. How you feel inside is how you treat others. "The daily challenge of dealing effectively with emotions is critical to the human condition because our brains are hard-wired to give emotions the upper hand," the authors write in

Emotional Intelligence 2.0[3]. "The communication between your emotional and rational 'brains' is the physical source of emotional intelligence."

Emotions get the upper hand in your brain. So, do you feel peace, or stress? Think of your mind as a computer desktop. Is it cluttered or well-ordered? What's it littered with?

If you've got negative, judgmental icons, replace them with positive emojis on your mental desktop. That inner critic we all have can be stressful when it keeps piping all its negative comments endlessly. Shift into happy face mode and your whole body will rejoice. Try it each morning before starting your day.

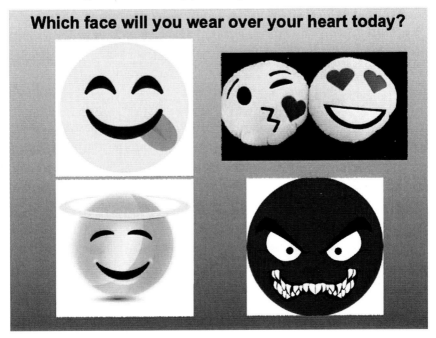

Which face will you wear over your heart today?

Listening to your favorite music can be a big help. It's how I got this book written. Music bypasses the judgmental brain to turn on your happy face.

Oxytocin is the hormone for relational bonding. You can get it through positive friendship (gripe sessions don't count), laughter, hugs, and healthy pleasures where safe. Newborns who don't get touched eventually die. Every one of us, regardless of age, has a baby inside needing that touch. Your mouth is also an organ for voicing your heart, singing, and connecting socially and spiritually.

Build quiet time into your day and week, off the hamster wheel, to nurture your mind as if it was a flower bed. Use that time to meditate or pray, walk in fresh air, hike outdoors (my favorite), dance, learn something new, or simply practice the tips in this book. In time, you'd feel calmer and kinder toward yourself and others, and less driven to eat.

Ground Yourself in the Present Moment

Getting a new dog to "heel" is far easier than getting your frantic mind to "sit." The "present moment" is a subtle yet powerful practice to redirect your stressed-out mind back to being yourself as a human.

I used to be really impatient waiting in line at the bank and grocery checkout or taking a number at the DMV or in restaurants. I've since grown a longer fuse by centering myself in the present moment the way you might sink into a super-plush sofa. A dear friend inspired me to take up mindful practice by calmly taking the time to hand-copy *Washing Dishes*[4], an essay by Thich Nhat Hanh, onto my notebook from the start to the final boarding call of her flight. I recommend you read it aloud like poetry, and savor each line like fine wine or dark chocolate:

> "To my mind, the idea that doing dishes is unpleasant can occur only when you aren't doing them. Once you are standing in front of the sink with your sleeves rolled up and your hands in the warm water, it is really quite pleasant. I enjoy taking my time with each dish, being fully aware of the dish, the water, and each movement of my hands. I know that if I hurry in order to eat dessert sooner, the time of washing dishes will be unpleasant and not worth living. That would be a pity, for each minute, each second of life is a miracle.

The dishes themselves and the fact that I am here washing them are miracles!

If I am incapable of washing dishes joyfully, if I want to finish them quickly so I can go and have dessert, I will be equally incapable of enjoying my dessert. With the fork in my hand, I will be thinking about what to do next, and the texture and the flavor of the dessert, together with the pleasure of eating, will be lost. I will always be dragged into the future, never able to live in the present moment.

Each thought, each action in the sunlight of awareness becomes sacred. In this light, no boundary exists between the sacred and the profane. I must confess it takes me a bit longer to do the dishes, but I live fully in every moment, and I am happy. Washing the dishes is at the same time a means and an end—that is, not only do we do the dishes in order to have clean dishes, we also do the dishes just to do the dishes, to live fully in each moment while washing them."

Thank you, Janice, for your generous sharing and for modeling how to stay in the present moment. To me, *Washing Dishes* evokes appreciation and gratitude, and inner peace by silencing my inner critic's incessant blabber.

This moment here and now is a miracle; so is the joy of that awareness.

If you crave peace and calm, look inward and take up mindful practice. "The primary roots of anger are in ourselves," Hanh writes in *Peace Is Every Step*[5]. "Our environment and other people are only secondary."

With the frantic mind put in its place, let's go to the yummy part— eating!

Chapter 23

Baby Steps Toward Your Holistic Mouth Style

"Overall health can be assured through a nutrient-dense diet, a robust gut microbiome, and an enhanced immune system."

~ Dr. Alvin Danenberg,
Is Your Gut Killing You?

The phone rang one day just as I was about to take a break from writing and enjoy a toasted orange-cranberry scone coated with ghee. The call was to fix to a silly bureaucratic request, and it frustrated me with endless "please hold" messages between transfers. During that time, I ate my scone in a huff—without tasting its rich flavor or experiencing the crunching pleasure.

What had happened? I allowed the call to turn on mindless eating to cope with stress. We all have our own "buttons" that can set us off to irrational choices. This awareness is a good start to adopt Holistic

Mouth Style. This a growth process that will continue with ups and downs for some time until you are in *total* control of your mind and mouth.

Adventures in Good Health Keeping™

Do you take care of business or chores while you eat? Eating without "the sunlight of awareness" amounts to using your mouth as a mechanical food processor set to high speed.

Do you watch TV or stare at your phone? Eating while multitasking leads all too easily to overeating and all its consequences. Being mindful is just one facet of Holistic Mouth Style. The rest includes how fast you eat and how much, in addition to what you eat.

Adopting Holistic Mouth Style means keeping the good in your current habits, dropping the bad, and finding healthier alternatives. "Then, what's left to eat?" Patients often ask after we talk about snoring causes and nasal congestion sources: dairy, wheat/gluten, sugar, eggs, soy, and others.

The short answer is plenty! Just add variety to your usual fare. This is America, where we have lots more to choose from than you can learn! Breakfast can be more than eggs and toast, and dinner does not have to be just meat and potatoes.

Try this new mindset: Make tasting healthier, slow foods an adventure in good health-keeping.

Variety and Balance

The longer answer to "What's left to eat?" is variety and balance. Just as cross-training is a key to superior sports performance, variety and balance is basic to thriving health.

Variety here doesn't mean different brands of packaged, prefab foods. Burgers and fries from different fast-food chains is not variety! As

Dr. Weston Price, DDS, wrote in his landmark book *Nutrition and Physical Degeneration*[2]:

> "We cannot distort and rob the foods without serious injury. Our modern process of robbing the natural foods for convenience of gain completely thwarts Nature's inviolable program…I know of no problem so important in our modern civilization as the finding of the reason for this, and the elimination of the cause of error."

Variety means eating foods with different colors, spices, and international cuisines. Guacamole, hummus, and sushi are good examples. Take a tour in an Asian or farmer's market with a knowledgeable friend to see what else out there has supported billions of people for eons. For some folks, this requires a serious new software install, but your brain is very capable of change if your mind is open.

From my neighborhood markets, I've had herring marinated with dill and onions in vinegar with warm millet porridge for breakfast, and avocado toast with sardines for a fast-break lunch. My dinner favorites include purple cabbage in spare-rib soup, and seaweed in fish broth for dinner—not every day, but periodically, for variety and balance. They combine to enrich my gut microbiome and help my body thrive inside and out.

Nourishing Traditions: Why Eat This Way?

Dr. Price extensively researched how modern processed diets affect the development of the jaws and teeth. "Probably the most indelible impression that is left by my investigations among primitive races," he wrote in *Nutrition and Physical Degeneration,* "is that which came from examining 1276 skulls of the people who had been buried hundreds of years ago along the Pacific coast of Peru and in the high Andean Plateau, without finding a single skull with the typical marked narrowing of the face and dental arches that afflict a considerable proportion not only of the residents in modernized districts in Peru, but in most of the United States and many communities of Europe today."

Nor did those skulls show signs of decay, another byproduct of modern processed diets. To regain the right state of overall health, Dr. Price concluded, "we would need to return to the use of natural foods which provides the entire assortment of the body-building and repaired food factors. Nature has put these foods up in the packages containing the combination of minerals and other factors that are essential for nourishing the various organs."

Dr. Price accurately predicted many of the health troubles facing Americans today. I have found jaw underdevelopment to be a root cause of many medical, dental, and mood symptoms, as well as a leading indicator of sleep apnea.

Non-GMO foods grown in unpolluted fields and unadulterated by factory processing are a crucial part of the solution. To keep Dr. Price's work alive, Sally Fallon founded the Weston A. Price Foundation[3] and co-authored *Nourishing Traditions* with Mary G. Enig, PhD. Both are valuable resources for using natural foods to bring out the best whole-body health and optimal cranial-dental development.

Bone broth and fish stew are among my favorites for building bone and thriving health. Here's an excerpt from *Nourishing Traditions*[4]:

> "A lamentable outcome of our modern meat processing techniques and our hurry-up throwaway lifestyle has been a decline in the use of meat, chicken, and fish stocks... Meat and fish stocks are used almost universally in traditional cuisines—French, Italian, Chinese, Japanese, African, South American, Middle Eastern and Russian; but the use of homemade meat broths to produce nourishing and flavorful soups and sauces has almost completely disappeared from the American culinary tradition.

Properly prepared, meat stocks are extremely nutritious, containing the minerals of bone, cartilage, marrow and vegetables as electrolytes in a form that is easy to assimilate. Acidic wine or vinegar added during cooking helps to draw minerals, particularly calcium, magnesium and potassium, into the broth. Dr. Francis Pottenger, author of *Pottenger's Cats*[5] as well as articles on the benefits of gelatin in broth, taught that the stockpot is the most important piece of equipment to have in one's kitchen."

Notice how variety is built into bone broth as a timeless staple across the world. "The main goal is to get you to see food differently, which will help you eat healthily for life," writes Australian dentist Dr. Steven Lin in *The Dental Diet*[6]. Indeed, variety expands your nutrients and broadens your taste experience, which is one of life's greatest treats!

Power Breakfast Without Eggs or Coffee

Without eggs, what's left to eat for breakfast? That was my challenge after I had tested sensitive to both egg whites and yolks—I had been feeling bloated after meals more and more. (Yes, it happens to doctors, too.) Now, I had to eat differently—get creative. Variety was, and will always be, the answer.

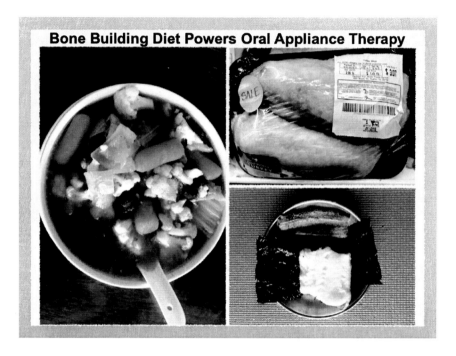

Bone Building Diet Powers Oral Appliance Therapy

Consider what I had this Saturday morning: turkey and vegetable stew with some sea bass broiled in my toaster oven for protein, and an organic chocolate green smoothie to sip throughout the day, sustaining me until dinner.

The stew was easy, made before going to bed the night before. I simply put two turkey wings and baby carrots into the bottom of my steamer pot, to which I added chopped onions, cauliflower, and water. Twenty minutes after pushing the "on" button, it was done. I cooked it twice to "milk" more minerals out of the ingredients. The broth is always the best part. Then comes the veggies!

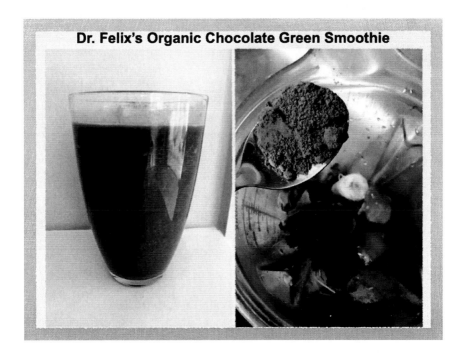

Dr. Felix's Organic Chocolate Green Smoothie

The smoothie was just as easy, made fresh that morning. I just blended up some arugula, avocado, cocoa powder, carrots, celery, banana, and tomato. Yummy, nutritious, and well worth a try! No coffee or dark chocolate needed to fuel me through my day—and my body loved it, as the blood sugar numbers show!

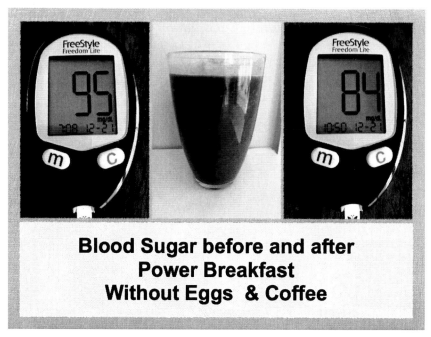

**Blood Sugar before and after
Power Breakfast
Without Eggs & Coffee**

100 is the lower threshold for pre-diabetes.

Another breakfast option without eggs, and gluten- and dairy-free, is oatmeal and bone broth. To make this, pre-soak walnuts (Goji berries optional) and glyphosate-free oatmeal separately in the morning. In the evening, place the soaked ingredients in a slow cooker, add filtered water, and plug it in so it cooks overnight. A delicious hot cereal will be waiting for you in the morning. Add a few tablespoons of bone broth (but no sugar) for a hearty breakfast. Thank you, Jasmine Ma :-)

Baked fish can also make a fine breakfast—especially a fatty fish such as wild salmon, turbot, or porgy. Not only do you get a good dose of protein, but healthy oils. Baked with a drop of lemon essential oil and paired with toasted seaweed, fish makes a top-notch breakfast to support your gut, brain, heart, and thyroid. Choose your fish wisely because of mercury in seafood[7].

I'm not a fan of processed foods, but I do fall back on canned sardines (in marinara sauce) paired with arugula or endive in a crunch.

Delicious, Nutritious, Easy, Versatile, and Healing

Bone broth and smoothies are my twin "turbo chargers" of a bone-building diet to go with epigenetic oral appliance therapy. They are also great for osseo-integration, the union of dental implants to jawbone after surgery. They are delicious, nutritious, easy, versatile, low-cost, and healing.

Smoothies provide rich antioxidants and vitamins and bioflavonoids from fresh greens and fruits. Bone broth supplies the minerals and proteins—in the form of gelatin—that your body can use to renew itself to stay young. According to Amy Myers, MD[8], gelatin—like collagen—helps "repair a leaky gut[9]."

Given the proteins, minerals, and vitamin C from bone broth and green smoothies, your body knows how to renew joints and ligament and grow jaws to widen airway for you to stay young inside and out.

"Aside from aging, the top reason people don't have enough collagen is poor diet," says Dr. Elizabeth Bradley, MD, Medical Director of Cleveland Clinic's Center for Functional Medicine[10]. "Your body can't make collagen if it doesn't have the necessary elements." Wrinkles on the face reflect collagen deficiency.

Bone broth is amenable to variety. You can use the carcass of half-eaten chicken, oxtails, ribs, pork knuckles, or lamb or beef shank, provided they are pasture-raised. You can add ingredients like onions, mushrooms, tomatoes, and spices for endless variety and consistent balance. Susan Brady[11], MPT, is an expert on bone health who provides an excellent video on bone broth[12].

Fish stock is the seafood version of bone broth, and it's just as tasty in its own way. Try a whole, gutted sea bass or croaker boiled for 4 to 7 minutes (size matters) in fresh ginger and scallion and leeks. You'll find plenty of basics and variations in *Nourishing Traditions Cookbook*. Ask your doctor if you should take chlorella to bind organic mercury in sea food.

Green smoothies are similarly versatile, so you can incorporate fruits and vegetables as they come in season. Think of it as making your own vitamins, minerals, and fiber supplements at home. I start with a base of arugula, adding a stalk of celery, a small tomato, and a few sprouts of any kind that I have on hand. To this, I add Brazil nuts[13] (rich in selenium, important in reproductive and immune health) or walnuts[14] (rich in omega-3 fats, good for heart and immune health) pre-soaked overnight, along with in-season fruits such as blueberries or watermelon.

Beware of overdoing the sweet fruits, especially if you need to regulate your blood sugar. Half a normal-sized banana is plenty for me. Unsweetened cocoa powder is optional, but it's a winner in combination with raspberry and avocado—thank you, Lisa Jackson, RN, AFMC :-)

Guidance from a nutritional or medical professional is important if you have pre-diabetes, diabetes, autoimmune disease, cancer, or chronic pain. Again, talk to them to get your thyroid, adrenals, and sex hormones balanced and sleep and airway restored for your self-regulation to work.

Dinner Without Meat and Potatoes

For Americans, dinner without meat and potatoes is as unimaginable as breakfast without eggs. Why not check out the global cuisines for variety?

An easy dinner I like is mushroom, celery, and garlic stir fry. Season to taste and you won't miss the meat at all on meatless Mondays. If the ingredients are fresh and sensibly prepared, you cannot go wrong. Add variety with imagination and trials. Share informal home-cooking ideas with friends and co-workers.

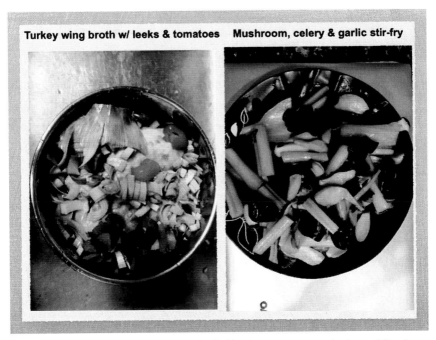

Turkey wing broth w/ leeks & tomatoes   **Mushroom, celery & garlic stir-fry**

Prep time for turkey wing broth (left): 4 minutes; cook time: 18 minutes in steamer. Prep and cook time for stir-fry (right): 7 minutes.

Another home-cooking favorite is meatball vegetable soup. Just blend ground turkey or chicken with finely chopped dill, mushrooms, and water chestnuts. Mash fresh tomato into a paste (use a blender set to low). Toss them into bone broth with some spinach or napa cabbage, and season to taste with salt and a touch of toasted sesame oil—"YUMMY!"

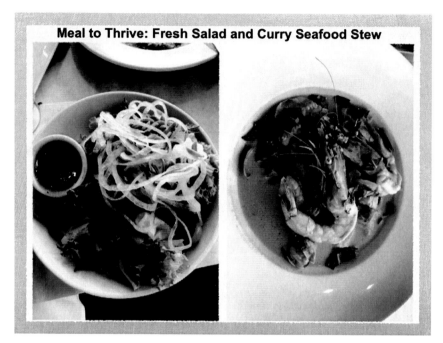

Meal to Thrive: Fresh Salad and Curry Seafood Stew

Lunch in Honolulu. Thank you, Auntie SuFang!

Variety also means that you don't have to do the same bone broth and green smoothies every day. Try a seafood curry/tomato stew. Add your pick of shrimp, scallops, clams, mussels, or fish to leeks, garlic, and onions with tomatoes or curry. With a side salad, this is an iodine-rich combination that supports your thyroid-driven functions on energy, temperature, and immunity.

Holistic Mouth Style Starters

1. Bone broth and green smoothies are the twin turbochargers to thriving health. Home cooking using whole foods from scratch (grandma-style) delivers TLC, variety, and balance to your body.
2. Eat and live as if you have pre-diabetes and high blood pressure. Consult with your doctor. Monitoring them yourself at home regularly is smart proactive personal care.
3. Put your caring into your healthcare. Regularly monitor blood sugar as a marker of your inflammation and degeneration. Stay away from the guardrails to avoid blindness, black toes, foot amputation, and kidney disease.
4. Learn to see cooking at home not as a chore, but as a blessing, just like *Washing Dishes*. Not only do we cook at home to make healthy food yummy, but we also enjoy eating each mouthful just to live fully in each moment.

Chapter 24

How to Eat and Thrive

"Our diet is rich in fresh fruits and vegetables, eat-en in-season only. We ate lots of fish and lamb that have never had any injections. Our way of life is a light breakfast between 7 and 9 am, a full lunch between 1 and 3 pm with a 20-minute siesta, a light dinner between 7 and 9 pm, and in bed by midnight. The average lifespan is about 95-100."

~ Maria from Spain's Catalan region,
excerpt from *Early Sirens*[1]

How does your lifestyle and mouth Style compare to the Mediterranean described above? Eating is a complex interplay involving all 12 cranial nerves connecting the gut with the brain and Mother Earth. Eating on the run, while multitasking, and under pressure with regularity is a recipe for indigestion and inflammation.

Mediterranean Diet: Food, Pace, Atmosphere

The Mediterranean diet is not just the foods on the plate. It's also a pace and atmosphere more compatible with health building. It feels like a Sunday stroll, not an all-out sprint.

The Mediterranean lifestyle includes going Yin: kinder, gentler, with a midday break, sunshine in the heart, and Mother Earth in the gut. We can bring this mindset and practice into our daily living, starting with Holistic Mouth Style.

I recommend you read the following steps *slowly*, at the Mediterranean pace, to let the points sink in, and then practice until they become habits. Speed reading here means little or no sustainable change in your old eating pattern.

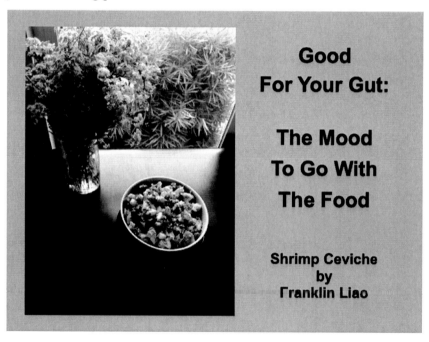

Good For Your Gut:

The Mood To Go With The Food

Shrimp Ceviche
by
Franklin Liao

Before you open your mouth, pause, and:

♦ **Know *why*.** Why are you eating this or drinking that? Are you feeling physically hungry, escaping some mental stress, or eating just because it's noon? Are you about to give your gut more abuse, or TLC? With practice, this will become second nature and less necessary.

♦ **Check your mood and stress level.** Are you too worked up for your Vagus Nerve to digest your healthy food? Is your "tail" pinched? Are you eating and drinking to escape stress? Take a breath, close your eyes if you can, and see if your old stress eating pattern has you in its grip.

♦ **Dial down your stress.** Turning on your favorite relaxing music can help. Or humming a song to yourself. Or saying grace and meaning it. Dial into gratitude—for the maker and growers of this food, your servers, your host, and for the food itself. Tell them you appreciate their work and the occasion. If you are by yourself, appreciate what your body does for you each and every day.

♦ **Downsize.** Use a lunch plate or fill your bowl to two-thirds full, or dinner plate to lunch size. Make it necessary to get up for seconds and see for yourself that you can eat right and feel happy by practicing the next steps.

Fuel To Thrive: Arugula Salad, Celery with Sardine

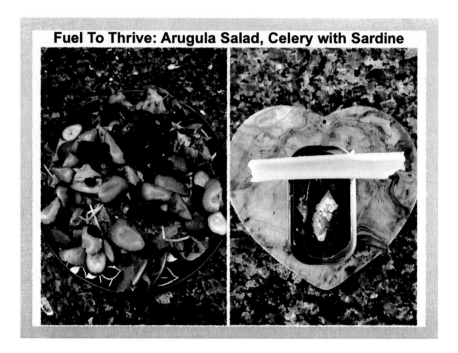

- **Digging in:** with the TV and smartphone turned off, and peace and quiet all around…

- **Be Present.** Take in the sight of the dish and the aroma of your meal to get your digestive juices flowing. Reflect on how it was made and brought to you before your first bite. Anticipate the flavors and textures of this dish/plate. Savor that first bite as if it were your first kiss all over again. It takes just a breath or two.

- **Compose each mouthful.** Mine is usually 90% greens/vegetables and 10% protein. Keep refined carbs down if you are watching your weight. Check with your HCPs. If you're susceptible to bloating or gas, or if you tend to feel tired after meals, consider Donna Gates' Food Combining Principles[2]: "enjoy protein with non-starchy land and/or sea vegetables… It is not ideal to eat animal protein and a starchy vegetable/grain at the same meal." This may explain why all-American fares like burgers and fries, or steak and potatoes, may not feel agreeable to your gut.

- **Slowly chew your food into liquids.** This will take lots of practice. The outcome is a gift for life you give yourself.

  - Allow time for food to mingle with your saliva fully to fully luxuriate in having delicious yet healthy food in your mouth.
  - Chew and mix them over and over, and don't swallow until you have chewed your food into liquids.
  - Pretend you are getting paid by the seconds you can keep food in your mouth.
  - Pause for the strong sensation in your mouth to subside before you reload.

Drop the obligation of finishing your plate until you have mastered these steps. Desserts left uneaten is a win, not a loss.

All the slow chewing and savoring allows time for your Vagus to signal to your brain that it's full. It's that simple to stop overeating.

How Much Is Enough?

If you're starved, one bite is never enough. But are ten bites enough? A thousand? How do you know how much food is enough for your health?

"More is better" is a recipe for disaster when it comes to your health. Is a supersized portion at the regular-sized price a good deal for your gut and arteries? How about the endless refills of sugary sodas? More likely, your gut would groan, "Oh, no! That mouth is piling it on again!"

So, what's a healthier way? "Enough" is a magic world, and it has been beautifully described by Joe Dominguez and Vicki Robin in *Your Money or Your Life*[3]:

> "Part of the secret to life, it would seem, comes from identifying for yourself that point of maximum fulfillment. There is a name for that point of Fulfillment Curve… The word is Enough.

At the peak of the Fulfillment Curve, we have enough. Enough for our survival. Enough comforts. And even enough little 'luxuries.' We have everything we need. There is nothing extra to weigh us down, distract, or distress us…

Enough is a fearless place. A trusting place, an honest and self-observing place. It's appreciating and fully enjoying what money brings into your life."

Enough shows up only when you slow down your mouth enough. Wolfing down or distracted eating leaves you with distention and aftermath. With guidance, attention, and practice, you will feel this subtle yet unmistakable message from your gut to your brain. That works only when your mind is consciously tuning into the feedback from your gut, not when it's elsewhere.

Observe the next time you eat with a group: How fast do people eat? How many gobble their food or savor it? Do they drink ice-cold beverages? When they're done, do they say, "I overdid it" or "That was perfect"? If children are present, notice how clearly they know they've had enough, and how they insist on not one bite more.

Enough is that happy balance between feeding your hunger and hurting your health with overfeeding. No expert can tell you where "enough" is, only your own gut. Enough is a narrow zone of five to six mouthfuls, in my experience.

Stopping at "Just right"

"Just right" is the apex of the fulfillment curve in Holistic Mouth Style. "Just right" is literally a gut feeling relayed to the brain— one you have had all along, except you've missed it while eating distracted.

With attention and practice, you will understand "Just right" as a precise point—a sweet spot accurate to that one mouthful. I'm smiling as I write this, for I've just noticed that I left $7/8$ of my dark chocolate almond bark uneaten. I had sensed that I had reached

"Just right" and stopped. I'm satisfied and happy—and isn't that the whole point of conscious and purposeful eating?

Once learned, "Just right" works for all your treats and all meals. You, too, will marvel at just how much your old eating pattern over-consumed.

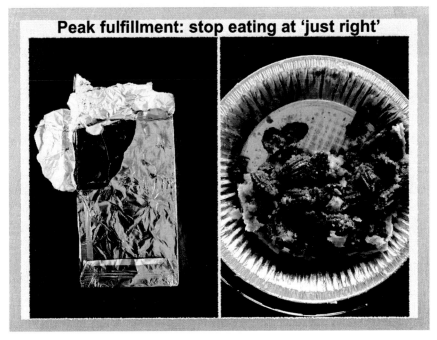

The amount of leftovers reflects burden avoided now and troubles saved later.

Stopping at "Just right" means less work for your gut, less burden for your joints to carry, and less inflammation all over. Savor your success and silently take a victory lap. Smile at yourself for stopping at "Just right," at the pleasure of enjoying another meal, at the leftovers on your plate, and at the people around you to spread the joy of eating in their company.

Try stopping at "Just right." You'd be surprised how much of that dark chocolate bar, cup of coffee, or plate of food is left compared to before, and therefore how much less exercise you'll need to work the excess off your waist.

Intermittent Fasting: Giving Your Gut a Break

"More and bigger" may be an endearing part of the American dream, but it's definitely not good for your health when it comes to eating! Today, survival depends on avoiding junk/fast/processed foods stripped of freshness and loaded with inflammatory health disruptors. What else can you do to counter the excess of added sugars, fats, salt, and preservatives in your face besides turning off your TV and smartphone?

Enter intermittent fasting. "Periodic fasting" has you eating one day then fasting the next. With "time-restricted fasting," you eat only during a limited window of time each day; for instance, eating during an 8-hour period then fasting for the remaining 16 hours of the day.

Life can be so simple during a fast—with no need to shop, nothing to prep, no dishes to wash, and no garbage to take out. A 3 to 5 day fast with Chi-Gong breathing and acupuncture support can be a powerful reset, in my experience. Be prepared to feel unwell from detoxing if you don't have professional support.

Fasting gives your gut a vacation—a chance to repair and recover. In 2017, the American Heart Association[4] found it could also "lead to a healthier lifestyle and cardiometabolic risk factor management." Whatever the method, fasting has a distinct health benefit, particularly for those of us on the other side of 39.

When I was young, "fasting" meant going hungry, and thus it was a repulsive idea to me. In my 60s, though, I've evolved to a two-meal day by listening to my body. If I wake up without feeling hungry, I don't eat until my stomach says to.

Intermittent fasting for me now means a late brunch and an early dinner, which allows for 16 to 18 hours of time-restricted fasting. Digestion is work requiring energy, which is why sleepiness often follows a big meal. I've come to see intermittent fasting as necessary downtime for my gut, appealing rather than repulsive.

Try making friends with "empty." Eat not by the clock, but by the signal from your gut. Just for the fun of it, try to see how long you can delay your next meal while still going on about your business. In time, and with patience, you'll discover you can live with 2 meals instead of 3 plus snacks. Then, you will be glad to have Empty as a friend under your belt. All this assumes that you are mindfully managing your stress and defusing your stress "detonators."

For more information, read *The Complete Guide to Fasting*[5] by Jason Fung, MD. If you decide to try it as an ongoing practice, be sure to consult with an experienced healthcare professional first.

Intermittent fasting means less work for your gut and more energy for your body. I've felt well and not grown a potbelly despite all the sedentary time required to write this book. As always, drink plenty of filtered mineral water or bone broth while fasting.

Chapter 25

Making Wellness Fun

*"I don't do drugs but if I think of sugar as a drug,
then I do them all day."*

~ Dr. Dawn Ewing

"I need another vacation to recover from this vacation!" Does that sound familiar? Also, "I'm on vacation, so I'll indulge now and diet after I get home"?

What's the point of going on vacation—to harm, or to restore yourself? Again, ask *why*. Having fun and enjoying life is the point of a vacation, staying home, and being alive. How can we make wellness fun anywhere? When the first draft of this book was done, I took my new Holistic Mouth Style with me on vacation to central Europe.

While I don't have a typical sweet tooth, I had come to enjoy coffee and pastry as "rocket fuel" to launch each reading/writing day. Combine that habit with too much sitting, flying to teach most weekends, and layoff from exercise from 2 mysterious sprain-like ankle injuries necessitating crutches, I had gained 10 pounds in 2 years.

The challenge was on: How could I have fun and still stay well?

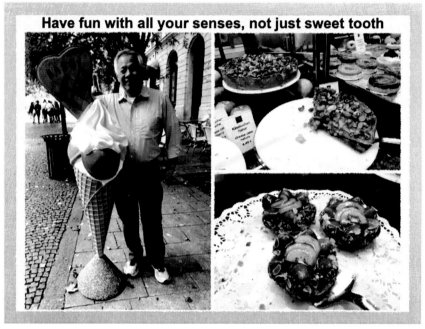

Have fun with all your senses, not just sweet tooth

I looked at all the enticing European desserts, smiled in appreciation, but was not reeled in by them as before—that's the point of getting "licensed to thrive."

I ate my fill, tried all kinds of local dishes and desserts, and came back without having gained extra pounds. My baby pot belly shrank by one belt notch upon my return, and I had no jet lag on Monday.

I perused and appreciated all the treats, picked a few, and stopped at "Just right" when I indulged. I enjoyed fully and returned healthier.

How did I do it? Just put my own advice into practice while on vacation—no magic needed, and no regret at all.

Vacationing with Holistic Mouth Style

"Vacate" means to leave a space empty. Vacation typically means leaving behind your work life and its stressors temporarily—a change of scenery while there, but no change in substance upon return except a few pounds heavier.

Isn't there a better way? Why not also leave behind old patterns like overeating while multitasking, mindless gobbling, and munching to escape?

While on vacation, I realized it's the best time to start habits. You are off the hamster-wheel—no bed or dinner to make, no chauffeuring the kids. That leaves lots of room on your mental desktop to focus on your Holistic Mouth Style.

Before going on vacation, I had researched the studies on sugar as an addictive substance (chapter 7). During vacation, my cognitive brain retained enough to defuse the knee-jerk reaction built into my primitive brain. The fancy pastries became artistic creations rather than irresistible hooks. Honestly, I hadn't expected such an about-face in my adventurous foodie personality!

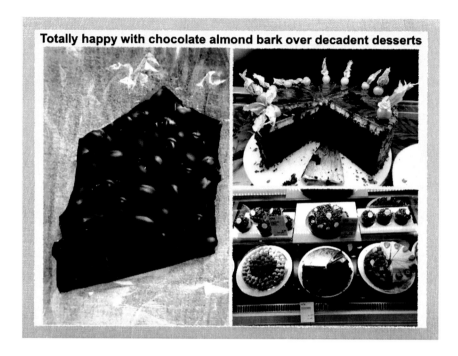

Totally happy with chocolate almond bark over decadent desserts

Stopping at "Just right" means there's room for dessert. After sharing a dinner of lamb shank, sauerkraut, and salad, I opted for a hunk of dark chocolate almond bark and thoroughly enjoyed that feeling of total contentment. (One of each would have been my choice before I started Holistic Mouth Style.) And I came back with more than just nice pictures.

Wellness doesn't have to take a back seat during vacations. Instead of sabotaging your health with over-consumption, you can build wellness into your vacation as a criterion for success.

Before you go on vacation or a long weekend at home, know the difference between tasting and over-indulging. Look beyond your pocketbook to consider what you can afford to inflict on your body and self-esteem, and how you'd want to feel upon your return.

Of course, you don't have to go on vacation to practice your Holistic Mouth Style. Consider a stay-cation, or vacation at home, and devote a whole day or long weekend to practice Holistic Mouth Style's baby steps in the previous chapter. It's fun to explore eating well (sustainably grown organic ingredients) and eating right (slower, kinder, more relaxed, thoroughly chewed, and stopping at "Just right"). It's also nourishing to cook at home from scratch spiritually to turn raw ingredients into tasty food, and to practice washing dishes mindfully.

Cooking at Home: Rewarding DIY in Minutes at Low, Low Costs

Every meal is an opportunity to either heal or harm your gut. That brings up my next point: cooking at home is far better for your health than eating out or getting delivery of standard/typical American fare. I too want to support restaurants and their workers, but I'm advocating for your gut and total health here.

As a foodie, I love and cherish farm-to-table restaurants that contribute to eating well, but they are few and far between. Most are in the mark-up business of buy-low and sell-high rather than cook organic whole foods from scratch. Their low margins require high efficiency, which means industrialized sauces from jugs and cans often high in health disruptors: MSG, preservatives, municipal tap water, and added salt, sugar, and fats, etc.

Restaurants rely on return customers to stay in business, and I understand fats, salts, and sugar are sure ways to appeal to prevailing palates that have been conditioned by Big Food and fast foods. Consider offering a few Smart Health-Keeping™ options to empower eating well and stand out in your community.

The surest way to eat healthy is to cook at home and make meals fresh in your own kitchen from whole foods carefully selected. Cooking at home declares, "I will take my health into my own hands, thank you, and I am taking control of what goes into my mouth."

The time devoted to home cooking is time well-spent. And you can often make several deliciously healthy meals at home for the cost of a single restaurant meal of doubtful health value.

My own favorites evolve all the time as I discover new dishes from different sources. Here's a 4-minute stir-fry. Heat up lard or ghee (clarified butter) in a pan, toss in chopped garlic, okra, and wooden ears (Chinese mushroom pre-soaked for 30 min), and season to taste (just a dash of salt for me). Bacon and scallops are optional. Thank you, Julie, for your home cooking and demo.

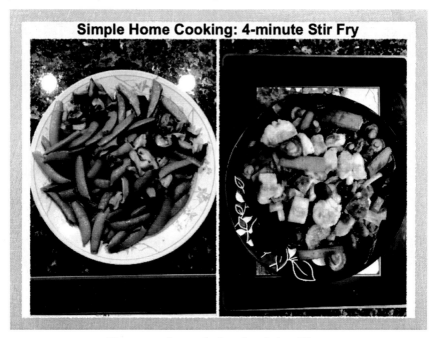

Home cooking dishes by Julie Chen.

Another is a Peruvian beef soup inspired by a local restaurant. It's easy to make:

1. Put beef ribs (or oxtail) in a crockpot to cook overnight or a pressure cooker for 30 minutes, then refrigerate so you can skim off most of the fat that has solidified on top.
2. Reheat, adding chopped carrots, cabbage, yucca, okra, leeks, and onions, etc.
3. Slow cook until the veggies are soft, and season to taste.

Remember to have fresh salad and/or green smoothies every day.

Excuses and Barriers

Trying new dishes, dropping old favorites, and eating slower is hard enough, and I can practically hear your objection: "Now you want me to cook?!" When change collides with entrenched habits, "I can't" invariably shows up.

The surest way to change how you eat, perhaps the only way, is to turn cooking at home into a treat. Remember your Declaration to Thrive? Now, ask yourself: "How can I achieve thriving health?" Daydreaming or complaining won't get you there, but cooking at home as described can.

Cooking at home is proactive wellness care of the highest order, along with sleep, exercise, and Yin/down time. It starts with your intention to be the best gardener for your gut health. Cooking for yourself means you have 100% control of how you eat and how well you eat—i.e., how much health disruptors get inside you. "Wellness" means having energy to keep your health and live your life, and that's well worth your time investment.

Another common excuse is that eating organic costs too much. "I can't afford it," many say. But can you afford the health damage from a steady stream of health disruptors undermining your gut health? You'll pay less to eat organic for a year than the hospital bills for an ICU stay or operating and recovery room use.

Your body keeps its own score, no matter how you rationalize in your head. Junk food makes junky body. Processed food favors obesity. Organic whole foods build health. Input leads to outcome—it's that simple.

So, stop the excuses and focus on what you *can* do. "Do not obsess over whether you can afford functional medicine. Obsess over eating what is recommended and eliminating what is harmful," suggests Dr. Terry Wahls[1]. "Obsess over what is in your control. And let go of what you cannot do or access."

Upgrading your mouth Style is worth obsessing over. And it's more economical than you may think. For instance, the wild caught Chilean sea bass in the image below seemed pricey at first: $17 for just over half a pound. Yet with a Holistic Mouth Style, I only needed 4 dollars' worth in combination with green smoothie and veggies in bone broth to reach "Just right." I don't need quite as much next time.

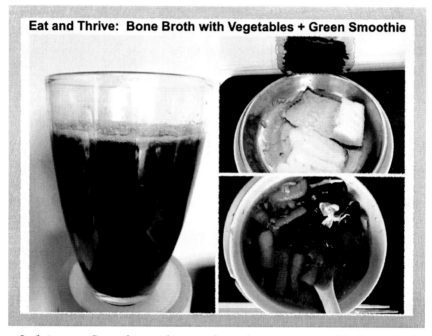

Eat and Thrive: Bone Broth with Vegetables + Green Smoothie

Left image: Smoothie with arugula, celery, tomatoes, blueberry, and banana.

Top right: Roasted seaweed, baked fish with lemon essential oil.

Lower right: Bone broth with carrots, onions, mushrooms, and a few shreds of chicken.

Foods such as raw veggie smoothies and cooked bone broth are easy, low-cost starters for those inexperienced in the kitchen. The longer you've been eating the standard American diet, the sooner and more dramatically you will feel the benefits of home cooking.

Thriving health requires nothing heroic, only an openness to go outside your habitual box to support your body with what it needs.

Try this simple low-cost exercise: Cut an organic celery stalk into inch-long pieces, and open a can of sardines in marinara sauce ($2.49 on sale) or whatever you have on hand (chili, smoked salmon, hummus, guacamole etc.). Put a piece of each into your mouth, chew mindfully to taste the blend of flavors fully. Don't swallow until you have chewed the celery into a pulp. I was full with one-third of the can left, and I fed my gut and fueled my brain to write this.

Besides feeling better, seeing the results of eating right is another great motivation for monitoring yourself, as discussed above. Take your blood sugar and blood pressure readings before bed, then again upon waking up, before you eat breakfast. Do this a few times, and you'll know how to tweak your mouth style in consultation with your HCP.

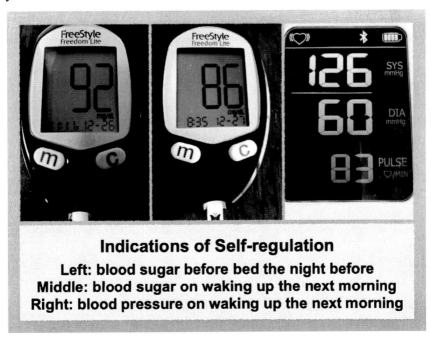

Indications of Self-regulation
Left: blood sugar before bed the night before
Middle: blood sugar on waking up the next morning
Right: blood pressure on waking up the next morning

Your energy will go up and your health will thrive as you sleep deep, eat well, and eat right. Depending on how far downhill your health is, good numbers may or may not show up right away. Keep your doctor informed. Don't fuss about daily fluctuations. The new trend line means more.

I recommend visiting or stating your personal Declaration to Thrive again now, and repeat it each morning. Then, enlist your family and friends as health-building buddies and your healthcare professionals as health-building partners.

Lessons from My Piano Lessons

My mom pawned her wedding jewelry to give me English and piano lessons when I was in grammar school in Taiwan. Fifty years later, I would see that acquiring new wellness skills is no different from learning a new sonata or next-level English. Thank you, Mom, and all my piano and English teachers.

Having to answer to a caring authority motivated me to practice. Without a teacher and a next lesson date, I'd be prone to slack off. The sooner I started practicing after each lesson, the more progress I made for the next lesson. You can start the baby steps of your new Holistic Mouth Style today, such as the celery chewing exercise.

This initial momentum is a strong self-motivator against procrastination. Progress from practice is the best reinforcement. I could feel it in my heart. Practice eventually becomes a habit and brings pleasure as its own reward.

Look for a caring health professional in your community who can be your "piano teacher" to monitor and support your Holistic Mouth Style, turning your patient-doctor relationship into a launching pad for Proactive Wellness Lifestyle.

Indeed, staying well is a bigger challenge than ever. As this 2015 Canadian study[2] says: "If you are 40 years old now, you'd have to eat even less and exercise more than if you were a 40-year old in 1971, to prevent gaining weight."

For that, you can thank the ubiquitous health disruptors baked into modern processed and fast foods. The same study concluded, "Weight management is actually much more complex than just 'energy in' versus 'energy out'…This is because our body weight is impacted by our lifestyle and environment, such as medication use, environmental pollutants, genetics, timing of food intake, stress, gut bacteria and even nighttime light exposure."

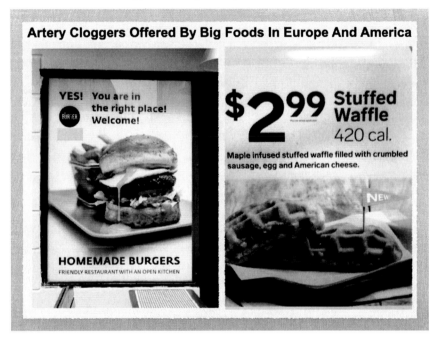

Adopting a Holistic Mouth Style and Proactive Wellness lifestyle is now more vital than ever, along with a well-developed set of jaws for good airway and sound sleep. We are already facing an epidemic of Alzheimer's disease, "the most common form of dementia," as this WebMD slideshow[3] puts it.

> "About a third of people 85 and older show signs of the disease...Dementia isn't a normal part of getting older. Except for age and genes, your odds of getting dementia go up with heart disease, diabetes, high cholesterol, high blood pressure, depression, obesity, stroke, poor sleep, smoking..."

What can you do proactively? This 2020 study Sleep Disturbance May Predict Rapid Cognitive Decline in AD[4] analyzed over 400 autopsy-confirmed Alzheimer's disease[5] (AD) patients, all of whom were initially cognitively intact: "Those who experienced nighttime behaviors (NTB: frequent awakenings during the night, rising too early in mornings, and/or taking an excessive number of daytime naps) at baseline had a significantly greater rate of cognitive decline than those without NTB."

Being proactive on Alzheimer's, obesity, sleep apnea, and inflammation reminds me of the inner game of tennis—seeing where your ball will go before you hit it with intention.

Eating for thriving health comes with its own "inner game," too. Do you want to end up in assisted living or a wheelchair, or independently living and dancing on your own feet all the way? Beating back inflammation and degeneration is the name of the healthcare game. Getting "licensed to thrive" is your best shot to win that match.

The only defense against Alzheimer's is a strong offense on airway-mouth-gut-brain connections to thrive health and bolster immunity. This does not mean eating celery every day. That exercise is just a training wheel to adopt Holistic Mouth Style.

You'll know Holistic Mouth Style has kicked in when you can notice old favorites are too sweet, too salty, or just plain too much, and you no longer crave or even want them. Your skin will look younger, your face will glow, and life is sweeter without the old sweet tooth screaming.

Postscript

I dropped 6 pounds in 6 months without feeling one bit deprived, just by following my own advice 80% of the time while writing this book. Weight loss is not the primary goal of *Licensed to Thrive*, but it can be a positive side benefit, depending on your compliance and preexisting conditions.

The primary purpose of Holistic Mouth Style is to build health and still have fun eating, socializing, and relating. I did just that when I went on my winter vacation after working night and day to submit this book's final draft to my editor. I now weigh just 5 pounds more than in dental school — not bad for someone who loves to eat after all these decades in America.

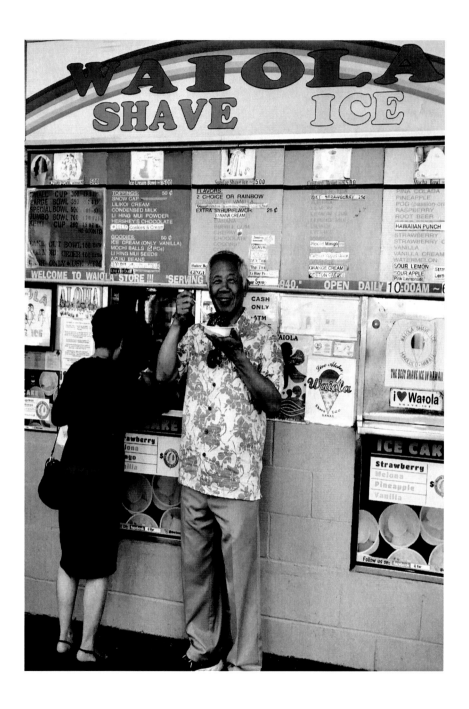

As you can see, I didn't hold back to enjoy a childhood favorite dessert treat from Taiwan. It's loaded with a lava of red azuki beans over a mound of shaved ice, topped with condensed milk—no guilt, even if it is hardly sound nutritionally.

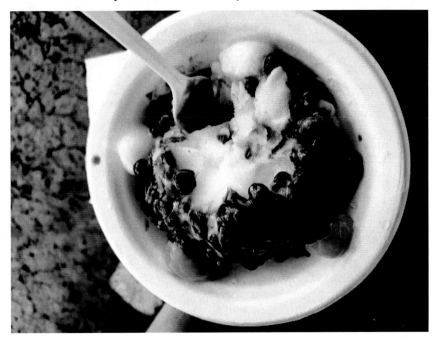

I could afford that treat then because my body could handle the sugar hit occasionally. My "homework" on mouth style reform had re-regulated my blood sugar to lower than pre-diabetes, and my potbelly has been shrinking. I now fit into my favorite pair of faded shorts from 25 years ago.

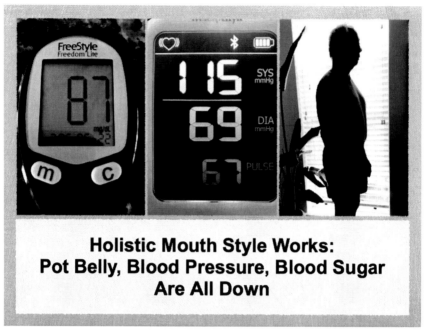

Holistic Mouth Style Works:
Pot Belly, Blood Pressure, Blood Sugar
Are All Down

Left to right: Fasting blood sugar, blood pressure on wake-up, and now, I just need to work on my writer's forward head posture.

Knowing HOW to eat has its rewards. The whole point of getting licensed to thrive is to build health, enjoy eating, and savor all the treats and goodies in America and this world. I wish you the same, and now you know how.

Afterword

"What have you done with the garden that was entrusted to you?"

~ Antonio Machado,
translated by Robert Bly

The cold hard truth is, the "cause of death" on your death certificate is likely driven by your mouth Structure and Style if you grew up in a first-world country or have lived in one for decades. Can you afford to keep your old mouth Style? What have you done with the mouth that was entrusted to you?

The great news is, you can take charge of your health by taking charge of your mouth—provided that you wake up to the need to change how you eat NOW. I hope *Licensed to Thrive* has primed you on the need for "driver's training" to steer your mouth toward thriving instead of failing health.

From Reading to Practice

Armchair reading is one thing, but putting advice into practice is quite another. Your challenge is to delete the old pattern of mindlessly eating from your brain and install a brand-new operating system called Holistic Mouth Style. Easier said than done. So, how do you start taking charge of your mouth? I recommend you do it in this order:

1. Make your Declaration to Thrive (chapter 15), tape a copy next to your bathroom mirror, and recite it each morning to keep yourself on task every day.

2. Make your Thriver's Priority List from these: impaired mouth structure, sleep hygiene, blood sugar and pressure monitoring, sitting and screen time, mental desk top, or holistic mouth style.

3. Talk with all your healthcare professionals (HCPs) about your Declaration to Thrive and enlist their support. Have your burden of health disruptors evaluated. Ask them to support you in monitoring your blood sugar and pressure at home, and keep them updated as you go.

4. Talk with your dentist or see an Airway-centered Mouth Doctor® (AMD) to assess your "6-foot tiger 3-foot cage." Identify oral contributions to all your symptoms checked off in Impaired Mouth Syndrome and get treated.

5. Once you have had your mouth Structure checked and addressed, start adopting Holistic Mouth Style. Focusing on diet and exercise without attending to your airway and sleep will fall short of optimal wellness.

An AMD (Airway-entered Mouth Doctor®) is not a speciality degree but a dentist who has taken additional training after dental school on connecting your mouth to head-neck alignment, airway, breathing, circulation, digestion, energy, and sleep, and knowing how to fix the defective links through WholeHealth Integration. AMDs are few and far between as of 2020. So, you may have to refer your own dentist to HolisticMouthSolutions.com. Here is an example:

> "Dear Dr. Liao: I just watched your outstanding interview with Suzie Senk, at the Holistic Sleep Summit[1]! You described my entire life!!! I have a narrow airway and choke and gasp awake. I wear a mouthguard to bring my lower jaw forward and I have a CPAP machine. They help, but I still don't sleep well.
>
> I'm 66 years old, and I would like to try your mouth device! Can tell us if there is a trained dentist in our area? I live in X-ville, Y-state. Is there an outstanding dentist here, who you trained? Or, I can come to you in Virginia…"

Looking ahead, there may be bumps in the road with mouth Style change. "You will feel crummy during sugar/carb withdrawal," Dr. Richard Jacoby advises in *Sugar Crush*. Dr. Steven Lin similarly notes in *The Dental Diet*: "the biggest challenges [patients] experienced were removing sugar from their diet and learning cooking techniques that were centuries old but new to them."

First Baby Steps

The journey to thriving health starts here, so please don't skip these initial steps:

- Make one little change one meal and one mouthful at a time. Follow my "recipe" on *how* to eat in chapter 5.3 point by point at each meal.
- Find a buddy for mutual support on this important and fun journey.
- DIY and cook at home using whole foods from scratch—it's TLC for your gut.
    - Go for variety, try something new, and go outside your usual box.
    - Make a bone broth, a green smoothie, or both (in their many variations) and see how your body responds.
    - Try sinking into mindfulness while chewing celery and washing dishes.
    - See how these steps and good sleep help with your sugar cravings.
- Do a "stay-cation" in your own home. Devote a quiet weekend or holiday when you can spend dedicated time to try out my suggestions above. Changing your mouth Style is harder in the grip of your daily grind.
- Stay engaged by subscribing to my blogs and newsletters, and share your home-cooking favorites and ancient wisdom from all cultures—please visit www.Licensed2Thrive.com.

- Learn new ways to enjoy healthy food tasty at home in 20 organized minutes with Cook2Thrive Chef Franklin—see Resources.

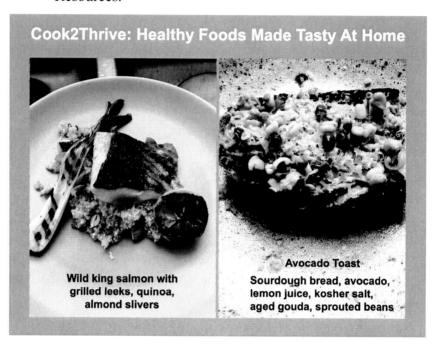

Cook2Thrive: Healthy Foods Made Tasty At Home

Wild king salmon with grilled leeks, quinoa, almond slivers

Avocado Toast
Sourdough bread, avocado, lemon juice, kosher salt, aged gouda, sprouted beans

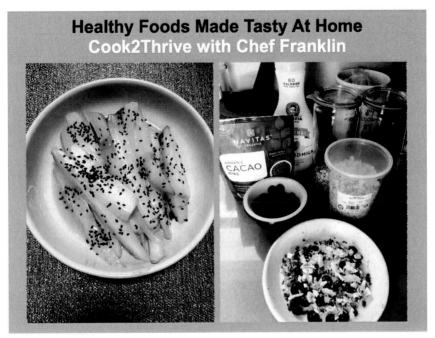

Healthy Foods Made Tasty At Home
Cook2Thrive with Chef Franklin

Above left: heirloom carrots, orange, and sesame. Right: overnight oats berry bowl.

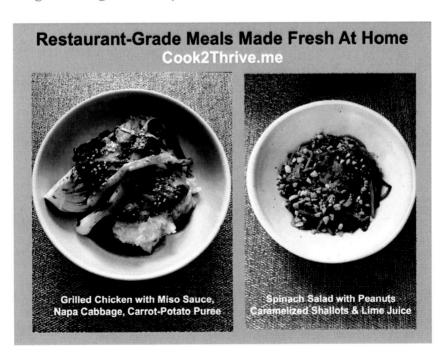

Restaurant-Grade Meals Made Fresh At Home
Cook2Thrive.me

Grilled Chicken with Miso Sauce, Napa Cabbage, Carrot-Potato Puree

Spinach Salad with Peanuts Caramelized Shallots & Lime Juice

Thriving health is something you build with personal care and keep up with practice and monitoring. Real change comes with guidance, monitoring, and support as you practice. Again, enlist your healthcare professionals' help.

Happy thriving!

If you are a dentist or healthcare professional, please see Afterword-2 next.

Afterword-2
For Healthcare Professionals

"Superior doctors treat diseases before symptoms appear, not after."

~ Nei Jing,
The Emperor's Internal Cannon of Chinese Medicine, 221 BC

A doctor's job is to alleviate symptoms *and* to find root-cause solutions to keep patients well. Impaired mouth Structure and Style are both root-cause problems.

An Airway-centered Mouth Doctor® (AMD) is trained in both mouth Structure and mouth Style correction. It is not an official degree from an accredited dental school, but a recognition of additional skillset to diagnose and treat Impaired Mouth Syndrome through rigorous continuing education. An AMD can help turn a structurally impaired mouth into a functional mouth to support airway and sleep, regardless of age. As a follow-up from Foreword for Healthcare Professionals, Miss Miller, age 67, emailed 4 weeks after starting her epigenetic oral appliance on her maxillary only:

> "The other big change from the oral appliance, I am sleeping better—longer and more deeply. So now I do not get exhausted at 1 or 2 pm. And because I am not exhausted, I am not overeating in an attempt to gain energy. And because I am not having the aching in my hip at night, I don't have the desire to eat something for comfort late in the night. I have lost a few pounds recently and am hoping and optimistic that I can continue to lose weight…
>
> Zero aching at night last night [3 days later]. Before oral appliance, the pain was there every night and I could only

sleep in 2-hour segments then awake a little bit and then sleep again through the night—so grateful...I have no pain in my hip except when I eat dairy—thank you for that."

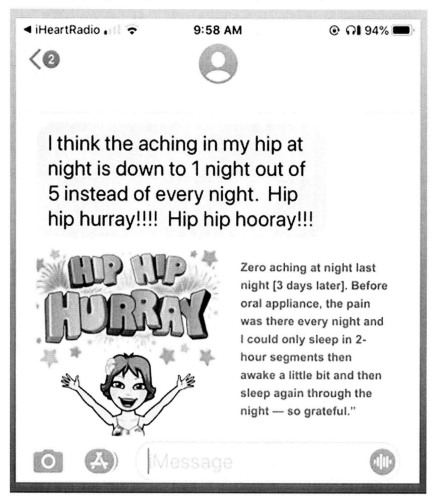

WholeHealth Integration means reaching across your lane and collaborating with other HCPs to deliver alignment, breathing, circulation, digestion, and energy (ABCDE) to all patients.

Non-dentist healthcare professionals (HCP): I invite you to visit HolisticMouthSolutions.com to discover how to become an Integrative Mouth Consultant and to find an AMD near you. Collaborating with an AMD can identify and remove oral contributions to amplify your clinical success.

An **Integrative Mouth Consultant** is a non-dentist HCP who can recognize Impaired Mouth Syndrome and work with an AMD. Becoming an Integrative Mouth Consultant is both beneficial and easy. Just start with online webinars and continue with working with an AMD on completing 2 cases.

A fully functional mouth is basic to physiology and homeostasis, but Impaired Mouth Syndrome was coined only in 2017. So, Holistic Mouth Solutions are not part of standard dentist training. Thus, AMDs are just starting to grow but are still few and far between. Consider referring your own dentist for AMD training to form new clinical cross-support and produce breakthrough outcomes as shown.

Dentists: The mouth is far more than teeth, and a dentist can become much more than driller and filler. Your patients are turning blue inside just waiting for you to liberate them from the tyranny of Impaired Mouth Syndrome.

Mandibular advancement device leaves out maxilla, the dominant arch affecting malocclusion, TMJD, nasal obstruction, and facial radiance. Every night guard is a missed opportunity to assess airway, improve sleep, fix pain, restore fatigue, and even save a life. The Earth is no longer flat, and the future of dentistry is in upgrading whole-body health by making the mouth work to support ABCDE. I invite you to start AMD training to elevate your game and reputation.

Take Care of Number One—You!

To better support all dentists who want to get started on their way to thriving personal health, I have started Dentists' Wellness Institute located in metro Washington DC, which is also open to all non-dentist HCPs as well.

The goal of this Wellness Institute is to help start healing the healer in you, as well as to provide a model for you to duplicate in your community. Over the years, I have built a WholeHealth team of like-minded, integrative HCPs to restore mind-body-mouth back to a functional whole.

Come with your Impaired Mouth Syndrome and leave with Holistic Mouth Solutions and a first-hand experience with WholeHealth Integration. Online consult is available as a first step—visit HolisticMouthSolutions.com/dentists-wellness-institute.

Happy thriving to you, too.

About the Author

Dr. Felix Liao is a thought leader and healthcare innovator who has restored the mouth back on the body as a vital organ for whole-body health and natural wellness. His WholeHealth philosophy advocates mind-body-mouth integration to produce breakthrough outcomes.

Among dentists, Dr. Liao is a leading airway-centered mouth doctor with recognized expertise in Impaired Mouth Syndrome and Holistic Mouth Solutions—two ground-breaking terms he coined in his bestselling books in 2017. In 2020, Dr. Liao has expanded Holistic Mouth Solutions to include both mouth Structure and Style to build vibrant health and innate immunity.

Six-Foot Tiger, Three-Foot Cage (6T3C) establishes deficient jaws with crowded teeth as a structural cause of choked airway, poor sleep, chronic pain and fatigue, and shows a structurally sound mouth is a natural solution to correct them painlessly while you sleep. *Early Sirens* identifies teeth grinding, TMJ, and problematic tongue for proactive treatment to avoid the costly complications described in 6T3C.

Dr. Liao's latest book, *Licensed to Thrive* advances new personal wellness care called Holistic Mouth Style: how to eat to grow bone and control metabolic diseases. It is the first book to integrate sound mouth structure with sensible eating style to build gut health and bolster innate immunity.

Clinically, Dr. Liao helps patients suffering from Impaired Mouth Syndrome with treatment plans to redevelop them into a sound infrastructure using epigenetic oral appliances and WholeHealth integration as needed to restore sleep, fix pain, and recharge energy.

Among dentists, Dr. Liao is a recognized Airway-centered Mouth Doctor® (AMD) and an expert on Impaired Mouth Syndrome's various medical, dental, and mood symptoms and how to fix them at the root-cause level.

Professionally, Dr. Liao is the Director of AMD Training Seminars® to help traditional drill-and-fill dentists become AMDs to deliver Holistic Mouth Solutions to patients. He is also the Founder of WholeHealth Integration Summits®.

Dr. Liao holds an engineering degree from Brown University, a DDS from Case School of Dental Medicine, Board Certification by the American Board of General Dentistry, Mastership in the Academy of General Dentistry, and Mastership in the International Academy of Biological Dentistry and Medicine (IABDM). He is a past president of IABDM.

Felix came to America from Taiwan at age 16 and has been a U.S. citizen since 1971. His personal interests include classical music, organic lifestyle, outdoors, hiking, swimming, dancing, science, world cuisine and culture, learning and teaching health-building skills, and adventures in making healthy food tasty.

Other Books by Dr. Felix Liao

Six-Foot Tiger, Three-Foot Cage: Take Charge of Your Health by Taking Charge of Your Mouth, 2017, Crescendo Publishing, LLC

Early Sirens: Critical Health Warnings and Holistic Mouth Solutions for Snoring, Teeth Grinding, Jaw Clicking, Chronic Pain, Fatigue, and More, 2017, Crescendo Publishing, LLC

Connect with the Author

Websites:	www.Licensed2Thrive.com
	www.HolisticMouthSolutions.com
	www.WholeHealthDentalCenter.com
Email:	DrFelixLiao@gmail.com
	DrFelix@HolisticMouthSolutions.com
Address:	7635 Leesburg Pike, Falls Church, Virginia 22043
Phone:	703-424-0322
Facebook:	https://www.facebook.com/
	wholehealthdentalcenter
YouTube:	https://www.youtube.com/user/WholeHealthDental
LinkedIn:	https://www.linkedin.com/company/
	HolisticMouthSolutions
Twitter:	https://twitter.com/wholehealthdds
Instagram:	https://www.instagram.com/
	theholisticmouthdoctor/

Acknowledgements

Excerpt(s) from *SALT SUGAR FAT: HOW THE FOOD GIANTS HOOKED US* by Michael Moss, copyright © 2013 by Michael Moss.
Used by permission of Random House, an imprint and division of Penguin Random House LLC. All rights reserved.

Excerpt(s) *THE ART OF RACING IN THE RAIN* by Garth Stein.
Copyright(c) 2008 by Bright White Light, LLC.
Used by permission of HarperCollins Publishers.

Excerpt(s) from *THE END OF OVEREATING: TAKING CONTROL OF THE INSATIABLE AMERICAN APPETITE*, by David A. Kessler, MD.
Used by permission of Random House, an imprint and division of Penguin Random House LLC. All rights reserved.

Excerpt(s) *THE PATH OF MINDFULNESS IN EVERYDAY LIFE* by Thich Nhat Hanh, copyright © 1991 by Thich Nhat Hanh.
Used by permission of Bantam Books, an imprint of Random House, a division of Penguin Random House LLC. All rights reserved.

Except(s) from *SUGAR CRUSH* by Richard Jacoby, Raquel Baldelomar. Copyright © 2015 by Richard P. Jacoby, D.P.M. Used by permission of HarperCollins Publishers.

Excerpt(s) from *CLEAN GUT* by Alejandro Junger, M.D.
Copyright© 2013 by Alejandro Junger, M.D.
Used by permission of HarperCollins Publishers.

Gratitude

I am grateful to all the patients who have contributed their stories and images to this book, and to all patients who have added to my experience through the years.

I am grateful, too, to all the instructors who have taught me—from my piano, English, and Chinese teachers in Taiwan to dental school, to post-graduate seminars in dentistry, medicine, and integrative health. I am grateful as well to all the authors quoted in this book, and the ones quoted in theirs.

I thank all my friends and colleagues who have encouraged and supported me through the years of writing this book: Jasmine Ma, my TCM teacher and inspiration; Dr. David Gruder, my all-around mentor and guide; my doctors and friends, Drs. George Yu, MD, Dr. Duyen Faria, MD, Dr. Judson Wall, DDS, and Dr. Cecilia Wu, MD; Lisa Verigin, my developmental editor; Jessie Martin, my office manager; Julie Chen for her home-cooking dishes and hospitality; Yang Liu for her invaluable assists with bibliography and permissions, and the world-class team at Crescendo Publishing.

Resources

A. Dentists: please visit www.HolisticMouthSolutions.com for
   - for AMD® Training,
   - Dentists Wellness Institute

B. Non-dentist Healthcare Professionals: please visit www.HolisticMouthSolutions.com for
   - Integrative Mouth Consultant Certification
   - One-to-One Consultation with Dr. Felix

C. Patient-Consumer Readers: please visit www.Licensed-2Thrive.com for:

   - Web-based training on how to develop your Holistic Mouth Style into personal wellness skill and continue as a habit,
   - Connecting with Chef Franklin at Cook2Thrive.me. He'll be your guide to make your home cooking healthy and tasty as recommended by Dr. Felix,
   - Sharing your own home-cooking that's deliciously healthy and yet simple enough for a fend-for-myself bachelor to make in about 20 minutes,
   - Video testimonials of patients in the order of their appearance in this book.

References

Introduction

1. MedicineNet, "Medical Definition of Innate Immunity," MedicineNet.com, July 16, 2020, https://www.medicinenet.com/script/main/art.asp?articlekey=26304.

2. Vighi G, Marcucci F, Sensi L, Di Cara G, Frati F., "Allergy and the gastrointestinal system," *Clin Exp Immunol.* 153, no. 1 (2008): 3-6, DOI: 10.1111/j.1365-2249.2008.03713.x.

3. Liao, F., *Six-Foot Tiger, Three-Foot Cage: Take Charge of Your Health by Taking Charge of Your Mouth,* Crescendo Publishing LLC (2017), Kindle Edition Available on Amazon: https://www.amazon.com/dp/B06X9ZDHTT/.

4. Liao, F., *Early Sirens: Critical Health Warnings & Holistic Mouth Solutions for Snoring, Teeth Grinding, Jaw Clicking, Chronic Pain, Fatigue, and More*, Crescendo Publishing LLC (2017), Kindle Edition Available on Amazon: https://www.amazon.com/dp/B0762S8G9B.

5. Besedovsky L, Lange T, Haack M., "The Sleep-Immune Crosstalk in Health and Disease," *Physiol Rev.* 99, no. 3 (2019):1325-1380, DOI:10.1152/physrev.00010.2018.

6. Bader GG, Kampe T, Tagdae T, Karlsson S, Blomqvist M., "Descriptive physiological data on a sleep bruxism population," *Sleep* (New York, N.Y., 1997): 982-990.

7. Weiss TM, Atanasov S, Calhoun KH., "The Association of Tongue Scalloping With Obstructive Sleep Apnea and Related Sleep Pathology," *Otolaryngology - Head and Neck Surgery* 133 (2005): 966-971.

8. Cariou B, Hadjadj S, Wargny M, et al., "Phenotypic characteristics and prognosis of inpatients with COVID-19 and diabetes: the CORONADO study," *Diabetologia* (2020).

9. Centers for Disease Control and Prevention (CDC), "Healthy Living," December 12, 2019, https://www.cdc.gov/widgets/healthyliving/index.html#bmicalculator.

10. Szumilas M., "Explaining odds ratios," *J Can Acad Child Adolesc Psychiatry* 19, no. 3 (2010): 227-229. [published correction appears in *J Can Acad Child Adolesc Psychiatry* 24, no. 1 (2015): 58].

11. Thorne, Deborah, Foohey, Pamela, Lawless, Robert M., and Porter, Katherine M., "Graying of U.S. Bankruptcy: Fallout from Life in a Risk Society," *Indiana Legal Studies Research Paper* No. 406, 2018, DOI: doi:10.2139/ssrn.3226574.

12. Stein G, *The Art of Racing in the Rain: A Novel*, Harper Perennial, 1st edition (May 22, 2018). Available on Amazon.

From Impaired Mouth Syndrome to Holistic Mouth Solutions

1. Indy Grit: https://indygrit.community/blog/2019/2/9/everybody-has-a-plan-until-they-get-punched-in-the-mouth; accessed October 27, 2020

2. Liao, F. Six-Foot Tiger, Three-Foot Cage: Take Charge of Your Health by Taking Charge of Your Mouth. Crescendo Publishing LLC; 2017. Available on Amazon.

Foreword for Healthcare Professionals on WholeHealth Integration

1. U.S. Department of Health and Human Services, *Oral Health in America: A Report of the Surgeon General*, U.S. Department of Health and Human Services, National Institute of Dental and Craniofacial Research, National Institutes of Health, Rockville, MD, 2000.

2. Schwartz D, Addy N, Levine M, Smith H., "Oral appliance therapy should be prescribed as a first-line therapy for OSA during the COVID-19 pandemic," *J Dent Sleep Med.* 7, no. 3 (2020).

3. American Academy of Sleep Medicine, *COVID-19: FAQs for Sleep Clinicians*, April 7, 2020, https://aasm.org/covid-19-resources/covid-19-faq/.

Chapter 1

1. Valderrama-Treviño AI, Barrera-Mera B, Ceballos-Villalva JC, Montalvo-Javé EE, "Hepatic Metastasis from Colorectal Cancer," *Euroasian J Hepatogastroenterol* 7, no. 2 (2017): 166-175, DOI: 10.5005/jp-journals-10018-1241.

2. Nieto FJ, Peppard PE, Young T, Finn L, Hla KM, Farré R., "Sleep-disordered breathing and cancer mortality: results from the Wisconsin Sleep Cohort Study." *Am J Respir Crit Care Med.* 186, no. 2 (2012): 190-194, DOI:10.1164/rccm.201201-0130OC.

3. Milner JJ, Beck MA, "The impact of obesity on the immune response to infection," *Proc Nutr Soc.* 71, no. 2 (2012): 298-306, DOI:10.1017/S0029665112000158.

4. Centers for Disease Control and Prevention (CDC), "People of Any Age with Underlying Medical Conditions," updated June 25, 2020; accessed July 16.

5. Centers for Disease Control and Prevention (CDC). *Adult Overweight and Obesity.* https://www.cdc.gov/obesity/adult/, page last reviewed: April 10, 2020; accessed June 28, 2020.

6. Ward ZJ, Bleich SN, Cradock AL, et al., "Projected U.S. State-Level Prevalence of Adult Obesity and Severe Obesity," *The New England Journal of Medicine* 381 (2019): 2440-2450.

7. Ellulu MS, Patimah I, Khaza'ai H, Rahmat A, Abed Y., "Obesity and inflammation: the linking mechanism and the complications," *Arch Med Sci.* 13, no. 4 (2017): 851-863, DOI: 10.5114/aoms.2016.58928.

8. Vighi G, Marcucci F, Sensi L, Di Cara G, Frati F., "Allergy and the gastrointestinal system," *Clin Exp Immunol.* 1 (2008): 3-6, DOI: 10.1111/j.1365-2249.2008.03713.x.

9. Louie J., "Obesity ups mortality risk for patients with H1N1," *Clin Infect Dis.* 52 (2011): 300-311.

10. Pinto JA, Ribeiro DK, Cavallini AF, Duarte C, Freitas GS, "Comorbidities Associated with Obstructive Sleep Apnea: a Retrospective Study," *Int Arch Otorhinolaryngol.* 20, no. 2 (2016): 145-150, DOI:10.1055/s-0036-1579546.

11. Chiang CL, Chen YT, Wang KL, et al., "Comorbidities and risk of mortality in patients with sleep apnea," *Ann Med.* 49, no. 5 (2017): 377-383, DOI:10.1080/07853890.2017.1282167.

12. Bonsignore, M.R., Baiamonte, P., Mazzuca, E., *et al.,* "Obstructive sleep apnea and comorbidities: a dangerous liaison," *Multidiscip Respir Med* 14, no. 8 (2019), DOI: https://doi.org/10.1186/s40248-019-0172-9.

Chapter 2

1. Hudgel DW, Patel SR, Ahasic AM, et al., "The Role of Weight Management in the Treatment of Adult Obstructive Sleep Apnea. An Official American Thoracic Society Clinical Practice Guideline," *American journal of respiratory and critical care medicine* 198 (2018): e70-e87.

2. Schwartz AR, Patil SP, Laffan AM, Polotsky V, Schneider H, Smith PL, "Obesity and obstructive sleep apnea: pathogenic mechanisms and therapeutic approaches," *Proc Am Thorac Soc.* 5, no. 2 (2008): 185-192, DOI: 10.1513/pats.200708-137MG.

3. Jenna's Case Videos: http://www.holisticmouthsolutions.com.

4. Belfor T, Advanced Faciodontics Seminars: https://drtheodorebelfor.com.

5. Singh GD, Griffin T, Cress SE, "Biomimetic Oral Appliance Therapy in Adults with Severe Obstructive Sleep Apnea," *J Sleep Disord Ther* 5 (2016):1, DOI: 10.4172/2167-0277.1000227.

6. Singh GD, Liao F., "Non-surgical improvement of the upper airway for sleep disordered breathing: 5 year follow up," *J OtolRhiol* 7 (2018), DOI: 10.4172/2324-8785-C3-014.

7. Weiss TM, Atanasov S, Calhoun KH, "The association of tongue scalloping with obstructive sleep apnea and related sleep pathology," *Otolaryngol Head Neck Surg.* 133, no. 6 (2005): 966-971, DOI: 10.1016/j.otohns.2005.07.018.

8. Hudgel DW, Patel SR, Ahasic AM, et al., "The Role of Weight Management in the Treatment of Adult Obstructive Sleep Apnea. An Official American Thoracic Society Clinical Practice Guideline," *American journal of respiratory and critical care medicine* 198 (2018): e70-e87.

9. Ramar K, et al, "Clinical Practice Guideline for the Treatment of Obstructive Sleep Apnea and Snoring with Oral Appliance Therapy: An update for 2015," *Journal of Clinical Sleep Medicine* 11, no. 7 (2015).

Chapter 3

1. Pessi T, Karhunen V, Karjalainen PP, et al., "Bacterial signatures in thrombus aspirates of patients with myocardial infarction," *Circulation* 127, no. 11 (2013): 1219-e6, DOI: 10.1161/CIRCULATIONA-HA.112.001254.

2. Lee IK, Kim HS, Bae JH, "Endothelial dysfunction: its relationship with acute hyperglycaemia and hyperlipidemia," *Int J Clin Pract Suppl.* 129 (2002): 59-64.

3. The International Academy of Biological Dentistry and Medicine (IABDM), https://iabdm.org/, IABDM Homepage, accessed June 28, 2020.

4. U.S. Department of Health and Human Services, *Oral Health in America: A Report of the Surgeon General*, U.S. Department of Health and Human Services, National Institute of Dental and Craniofacial Research, National Institutes of Health, Rockville, MD, 2000.

5. Ravnskov U. MD, *Ignore the Awkward: How Cholesterol Muths Are kept Alive.* CreateSpace Independent Publishing Platform (January 10, 2010). Available on Amazon.

6. Carlson R, Kenyon P, Yee M, *Death By Root Canal: Slow Blood Poisoning*, Honolulu: Smashwords Inc. (July 10, 2019).

7. Caplan DJ, et al, "The relationship between self-reported history of endodontic therapy and coronary heart disease in the Atherosclerosis Risk in Communities Study," *J Am Dent Assoc.* 140, no. 8 (2009): 1004–1012, PMID: 19654253.

8. Hernández Vigueras S, Donoso Zúñiga M, Jané-Salas E, et al., "Viruses in pulp and periapical inflammation: a review," *Odontology* 104, no. 2 (2016): 184-191, DOI:10.1007/s10266-015-0200-y.

9. Levy TE, MD, JD, *Hidden Epidemic: Silent Oral Infections Cause Most Heart Attacks and Breast Cancers,* MedFox Publishing (2017), Amazon: https://www.amazon.com/Hidden-Epidemic-Infections-Attacks-Cancers/dp/0983772878.

10. Danenberg A, DDS. *Is Your Gut Killing You? An in-depth guide on the connection between the gut, the mouth, chronic disease, and how to stay healthy,* www.drdanenberg.com, July 2020, Available on Amazon.

11. Levy TE, MD, JD. *Hidden Epidemic*, Amazon: https://www.amazon.com/Hidden-Epidemic-Infections-Attacks-Cancers/dp/0983772878.

Chapter 4

1. Cargill K, *The Psychology of Overeating.* Bloomsbury Academic (2015). Amazon: https://www.amazon.com/Psychology-Overeating-Food-Culture-Consumerism-ebook/dp/B014UXFZVQ.

2. Moss M, *Salt Sugar Fat: How the Food Giants Hooked Us,* Random House (2013). Available on Amazon.

3. Wilson, B., How ultra-processed food took over your shopping basket, *The Guardian*, Feb. 12, 2020, accessed June 28, 2020.

4. Junger A, MD. *Clean Gut: The Breakthrough Plan for Eliminating the Root Cause of Disease and Revolutionizing Your Health*, HarperOne, 1 edition (April 30, 2013). Available on Amazon.

5. Yong E., *I Contain Multitudes: The Microbes Within Us and a Grander View of Life*, Ecco, 1 edition (August 9, 2016). Available on Amazon.

6. Berg JM, Tymoczko JL, Stryer L, *Biochemistry*, 5th edition. New York: W H Freeman (2002). Chapter 17, The Citric Acid Cycle. Available from: https://www.ncbi.nlm.nih.gov/books/NBK21163/.

7. Cui J, Mao X, Olman V, Hastings PJ, Xu Y., "Hypoxia and miscoupling between reduced energy efficiency and signaling to cell proliferation drive cancer to grow increasingly faster," *J Mol Cell Biol.* 4, no. 3 (2012): 174-176, DOI:10.1093/jmcb/mjs017.

8. Mahdavinia M, Keshavarzian A, Tobin MC, Landay AL, Schleimer RP, "A comprehensive review of the nasal microbiome in chronic rhinosinusitis (CRS)," *Clin Exp Allergy* 46, no. 1 (2016): 21-41, DOI:10.1111/cea.12666.

9. Huang YJ, Marsland BJ, Bunyavanich S, et al., "The microbiome in allergic disease: Current understanding and future opportunities-2017," PRACTALL document of the American Academy of Allergy, Asthma & Immunology and the European Academy of Allergy and Clinical Immunology, *J Allergy Clin Immunol.* 139, no. 4 (2017): 1099-1110, DOI: 10.1016/j.jaci.2017.02.007.

10. Hrncirova L, Machova V, Trckova E, Krejsek J, Hrncir T, "Food Preservatives Induce *Proteobacteria* Dysbiosis in Human-Microbiota Associated *Nod2*-Deficient Mice," *Microorganisms* 7, no. 10 (2019): 383, DOI: 10.3390/microorganisms7100383.

11. Colquhoun J., "22 Additives And Preservatives To Avoid," *Food Matters*, Nov. 01, 2016, https://www.foodmatters.com/article/22-additives-and-preservatives-to-avoid.

12. Zinöcker MK, Lindseth IA, "The Western Diet-Microbiome-Host Interaction and Its Role in Metabolic Disease," *Nutrients* 10, no. 3 (2018): 365, DOI: 10.3390/nu10030365.

Chapter 5

1. Bischoff SC, Barbara G, Buurman W, et al., "Intestinal permeability—a new target for disease prevention and therapy," *BMC Gastroenterol* 14 (2014): 189, DOI: 10.1186/s12876-014-0189-7

2. Spritzler F., "Anti-Inflammatory Diet 101: How to Reduce Inflammation Naturally," *Healthline,* Dec. 13, 2018. https://www.healthline.com/nutrition/anti-inflammatory-diet-101.

3. Lustig R, MD, "Isocaloric fructose restriction and metabolic improvement in children with obesity and metabolic syndrome," *Obesity* (Silver Spring) 24, no. 2 (2016): 453–460, PMID: 26499447.

4. Spruss A, Kanuri G, Stahl C, Bischoff SC, Bergheim I, "Metformin protects against the development of fructose-induced steatosis in mice: role of the intestinal barrier function," *Lab Invest*. 92, no. 7 (2012): 1020-1032, DOI: 10.1038/labinvest.2012.75.

5. Tennant JL, *Healing is Voltage: The Handbook*, 3rd edition, CreateSpace Independent Publishing Platform. Available on Amazon: https://www.amazon.com/Healing-Voltage-Handbook-Jerry-Tennant/dp/1453649166.

6. Davidson K., "Should You Use Rapeseed Oil? Everything You Need to Know," *Healthline,* Oct. 30, 2019. https://www.healthline.com/nutrition/rapeseed-oil.

7. Borg K., "Physiopathological effects of rapeseed oil: a review," *Acta Med Scand Suppl*. 585 (1975): 5-13, DOI: 10.1111/j.0954-6820.1975.tb06554.x.

8. Aguila MB, Mandarim-de-Lacerda CA, "Numerical density of cardiac myocytes in aged rats fed a cholesterol-rich diet and a canola oil diet (n-3 fatty acid rich)," *Virchows Arch*. 434, no. 5 (1999): 451-453, DOI: 10.1007/s004280050365.

9. American Cancer Society, *Known and Probable Human Carcinogens*, https://www.cancer.org/cancer/cancer-causes/general-info/known-and-probable-human-carcinogens.html. Last Medical Review: May 17, 2019. Accessed June 28, 2020.

10. Vainio H., "Public health and evidence-informed policy-making: The case of a commonly used herbicide," *Scand J Work Environ Health*. 46, no. 1 (2020):105-109, DOI: 10.5271/sjweh.3851.

11. Samsel A, Seneff S., "Glyphosate, pathways to modern diseases II: Celiac sprue and gluten intolerance," *Interdiscip Toxicol*. 6, no. 4 (2013): 159-184, DOI: 10.2478/intox-2013-0026.

12. Myers, J.P., Antoniou, M.N., Blumberg, B. *et al.,* "Concerns over use of glyphosate-based herbicides and risks associated with exposures: a consensus statement," *Environ Health* 15 (2016): 19, DOI: https://doi.org/10.1186/s12940-016-0117-0.

13. Seneff S., "Glyphosate," *Learn True Health*, https://www.learntrue-health.com/glyphosate/. (n.d.) Accessed June 28, 2020.

Chapter 6

1. American Sleep and Breathing Academy (ASBA), https://asba.net/, ASBA Homepage. Accessed July 1, 2020.

2. Schwartz AR, Patil SP, Laffan AM, Polotsky V, Schneider H, Smith PL, "Obesity and obstructive sleep apnea: pathogenic mechanisms and therapeutic approaches," *Proc Am Thorac Soc.* 5, no. 2 (2008): 185-192, DOI: 10.1513/pats.200708-137MG.

3. Santos T, Drummond M, Botelho F., "Erectile dysfunction in obstructive sleep apnea syndrome—prevalence and determinants," *Revista portuguesa de pneumologia* 18 (2012): 64.

4. McNamara D., "Stroke Risk Tied to Diabetic Retinopathy May Not Be Modifiable Damian," *Medscape*, February 13, 2020. https://www.medscape.com/viewarticle/925223?src=wnl_edit_tpal&uac=175928D-V&impID=2279018&faf=1#vp_2.

5. Moore JX, Chaudhary N, Akinyemiju T., "Metabolic Syndrome Prevalence by Race/Ethnicity and Sex in the United States," National Health and Nutrition Examination Survey, 1988-2012, *Preventing chronic disease* 14 (2017): E24.

Chapter 7

1. Sanchez A, Reeser JL, Lau HS, et al., "Role of sugars in human neutrophilic phagocytosis," *The American journal of clinical nutrition* 26 (1973): 1180-1184.

2. Jacoby RP, *Sugar Crush: How to Reduce Inflammation, Reverse Nerve Damage, and Reclaim Good Health,* Harper Wave 2016, http://sugarcrushthebook.com.

3. Lenoir M, Serre F, Cantin L, Ahmed SH, "Intense sweetness surpasses cocaine reward," *PloS one* 2 (2007): e698.

4. Avena NM, Rada P, Hoebel BG, "Evidence for sugar addiction: behavioral and neurochemical effects of intermittent, excessive sugar intake," *Neurosci Biobehav Rev.* 32, no. 1 (2008): 20-39, DOI: 10.1016/j.neubiorev.2007.04.019.

5. Fuhrman J. Negative Impact of Sugar on the Brain, *Verywell Mind*, June 16, 2020, https://www.verywellmind.com/how-sugar-affects-the-brain-4065218.

6. Do MH, Lee E, Oh MJ, Kim Y, Park HY, "High-Glucose or -Fructose Diet Cause Changes of the Gut Microbiota and Metabolic Disorders in Mice without Body Weight Change," *Nutrients* 10, no. 6 (2018): 761, published 2018 Jun 13, DOI: 10.3390/nu10060761.

7. Gkogkolou P, Böhm M, "Advanced glycation end products: Key players in skin aging?" *Dermatoendocrinol* 4, no. 3 (2012): 259-270, DOI: 10.4161/derm.22028.

8. Neves D, "Advanced glycation end-products: a common pathway in diabetes and age-related erectile dysfunction," *Free Radic Res.* 47, no. 1 (2013): 49-69, DOI: 10.3109/10715762.2013.821701.

9. Aeberli I, Gerber PA, Hochuli M, et al., "Low to moderate sugar-sweetened beverage consumption impairs glucose and lipid metabolism and promotes inflammation in healthy young men: a randomized controlled trial," *Am J Clin Nutr.* 94, no. 2 (2011): 479-485, DOI: 10.3945/ajcn.111.013540.

10. Buyken AE, Flood V, Empson M, et al., "Carbohydrate nutrition and inflammatory disease mortality in older adults," *Am J Clin Nutr.* 92, no. 3 (2010): 634-643, DOI: 10.3945/ajcn.2010.29390.

11. Martin ET, Kaye KS, Knott C, et al., "Diabetes and Risk of Surgical Site Infection: A Systematic Review and Meta-analysis," *Infect Control Hosp Epidemiol.* 37, no. 1 (2016): 88-99, DOI: 10.1017/ice.2015.249.

12. WebMD. Slideshow: The Truth About Sugar Addiction, *WebMD*, April 7, 2020, https://www.webmd.com/diet/ss/slideshow-sugar-addiction.

13. Centers for Disease Control and Prevention (CDC), *Know Your Limit for Added Sugars*, https://www.cdc.gov/nutrition/data-statistics/know-your-limit-for-added-sugars.html.

14. McCulloch M., "Is Orange Juice Good or Bad for You?" *Healthline*, Dec 13, 2018, https://www.healthline.com/nutrition/orange-juice.

15. Ferdman RA., "Where people around the world eat the most sugar and fat," *The Washington Post*, Feb. 5, 2015, https://www.washingtonpost.com/news/wonk/wp/2015/02/05/where-people-around-the-world-eat-the-most-sugar-and-fat/.

16. Raatz SK, Johnson LK, Picklo MJ, "Consumption of Honey, Sucrose, and High-Fructose Corn Syrup Produces Similar Metabolic Effects in Glucose-Tolerant and -Intolerant Individuals," *J Nutr.* 145, no. 10 (2015): 2265-2272, DOI: 10.3945/jn.115.218016.

17. Goran M., Michael I, Goran Lab Homepage. http://www.goranlab.com/.

18. Walker RW, Ph.D, Dumke KA, M.S, Goran MI, Ph.D., "Fructose content in popular beverages made with and without high-fructose corn syrup," *Nutrition* 30 (2014): 928-935.

Chapter 8

1. Fung J MD, *The Diabetes Code: Prevent and Reverse Type 2 Diabetes Naturally*, Greystone Books, 1 edition (April 3, 2018). Available on Amazon.

2. Kalamut A. This Is Your Brain On Drugs - 80s Partnership For A Drug Free America. *YouTube*. https://www.youtube.com/watch?v=GOnEN-VylxPI&feature=youtu.be.

3. Moss M, *Salt Sugar Fat: How the Food Giants Hooked Us,* Random House (2013). Available on Amazon.

4. Lenoir M, Serre F, Cantin L, Ahmed SH, "Intense sweetness surpasses cocaine reward," *PLoS One* 2, no. 8 (2007): e698. Published 2007 Aug 1, DOI: 10.1371/journal.pone.0000698.

Chapter 9

5. Kessler DA, *The End of Overeating*, Rodale Books (2009). Amazon: https://www.amazon.com/End-Overeating-Insatiable-American-Appetite/dp/1605297852.

6. Wikipedia. Classical conditioning. *Wikipedia*. https://en.wikipedia. org/wiki/Classical_conditioning. Last edited on June 20, 2020. Accessed July 1, 2020.

Chapter 10

1. Cargill K, *The Psychology of Overeating*. Bloomsbury Academic (2015). Amazon: https://www.amazon.com/Psychology-Overeating-Food-Culture-Consumerism-ebook/dp/B014UXFZVQ.

2. Golin M. "Yearning to be stress-free: what aggravates Americans most?" *Prevention 3 (*1995): 74. http://search.ebscohost.com/login.aspx?direct=true&site=eds-live&db=edsgih&AN=edsgcl.16745796&custid=s6224580.

3. Antelman SM, Szechtman H, Chin P, Fisher AE., "Tail pinch-induced eating, gnawing and licking behavior in rats: dependence on the nigrostriatal dopamine system," *Brain Res*. 99, no. 2 (1975): 319-337, DOI: 10.1016/0006-8993(75)90032-3.

4. NPR/Robert Wood Johnson Foundation/Harvard School of Public Health, "The Burden of Stress in America," *Robert Wood Johnson Foundation*, July 7, 2014, https://www.rwjf.org/en/library/research/2014/07/the-burden-of-stress-in-america.html.

5. Centers for Disease Control and Prevention (CDC), *Healthy Living Widgets*, published December 12, 2019; accessed June 28, 2020. https://www.cdc.gov/widgets/healthyliving/index.html#bmicalculator.

6. World Health Organization (WHO), "Obesity and Overweight," accessed July 1, 2020, retrieved from https://www.who.int/dietphysicalactivity/media/en/gsfs_obesity.pdf.

7. Molina B., "More than 1 in 3 adults eat fast food on a given day, CDC survey finds," *USA TODAY*, Oct. 3, 2018. https://www.usatoday.com/story/news/nation-now/2018/10/03/americans-eat-fast-food-daily-cdc-survey/1507702002/.

8. UHN Staff, "Fast Food and Obesity: The Cold, Hard Facts," *University Health News*, Jan. 29, 2014, https://universityhealthnews.com/daily/nutrition/fast-food-and-obesity-the-cold-hard-facts/. Accessed July 1, 2020.

9. Knutson KL, Spiegel K, Penev P, Van Cauter E, "The metabolic consequences of sleep deprivation," *Sleep Med Rev.* 11, no. 3 (2007): 163-178, DOI: 10.1016/j.smrv.2007.01.002.

10. Layton J. "Is a lack of sleep making me fat?" n.d. https://science.howstuffworks.com/life/inside-the-mind/human-brain/sleep-obesity1.htm. Accessed July 1, 2020.

11. Kentish SJ, Frisby CL, Kennaway DJ, Wittert GA, Page AJ, "Circadian variation in gastric vagal afferent mechanosensitivity," *J Neurosci* 33, no. 49 (2013): 19238-19242, DOI: 10.1523/JNEUROSCI.3846-13.2013.

12. RightSleep, https://drgominak.com/, RightSleep Homepage, accessed June 28, 2020.

13. Gominak SC, Stumpf WE, "The world epidemic of sleep disorders is linked to vitamin D deficiency," *Med Hypotheses* 79, no. 2 (2012):132-135, DOI: 10.1016/j.mehy.2012.03.031.

14. Gominak S. "Vitamin D deficiency changes the intestinal microbiome reducing B vitamin production in the gut. The resulting lack of pantothenic acid adversely affects the immune system, producing a 'pro-inflammatory' state associated with atherosclerosis and autoimmunity," *Medical Hypotheses* 94 (2016): 103-107, DOI: 10.1016/j.mehy.2016.07.007.

Chapter 11

1. Junger A, MD, *Clean Gut: The Breakthrough Plan for Eliminating The Root Cause of Disease and Revolutionize Your Health*, HarperOne (2013). Available on Amazon.

2. Gregor MF, Hotamisligil GS, "Inflammatory mechanisms in obesity," *Annual review of immunology*, 29 (2011): 415-445.

Chapter 12

1. Chief Seattle, Web of Life, 1854. awaking.org: https://www.awakin.org/read/view.php?tid=345

2. Carroll L., "Low Levels of Environmental Pollutants May Slow Fetal Growth," *Medscape*, Dec. 31, 2017. https://www.medscape.com/viewarticle/923218?src=wnl_edit_tpal&uac=175928DV&impID=2230161&faf=1. Accessed July 1, 2020.

3. U.S. Geological Survey, "Pharmaceuticals in Water," n.d. USGS. https://www.usgs.gov/special-topic/water-science-school/science/pharmaceuticals-water?qt-science_center_objects=0#qt-science_center_objects. Accessed July 1, 2020.

4. Parker L., "Baby fish have started eating plastic. We haven't yet seen the consequences," *National Geographic*. Appeared in May 2019 issue. https://www.nationalgeographic.com/magazine/2019/05/microplastics-impact-on-fish-shown-in-pictures/. Accessed July 1, 2020.

5. Case J., "Through the Lens of a Microscope: How plastics are impacting our oceans," *National Geographic*. May 21, 2019. https://blog.nationalgeographic.org/2019/05/21/through-the-lens-of-a-microscope-how-plastics-are-impacting-our-oceans/?utm_source=ngs&utm_medium=email&utm_campaign=2019-julyenews&utm_content=-gen-dn. Accessed July 1, 2020.

6. The Plastics Pollutions Coalition, The Plastics Pollutions Coalition Homepage. https://www.plasticpollutioncoalition.org/. Accessed July 1, 2020.

7. President's Cancer Panel. *2008-2009 Annual Report: Reducing environmental cancer risk - what we can do now,* April 2010. https://deainfo.nci.nih.gov/advisory/pcp/annualreports/pcp08-09rpt/pcp_report_08-09_508.pdf. Accessed July 1, 2020.

8. Di Renzo GC, Conry JA, Blake J, et al., "International Federation of Gynecology and Obstetrics opinion on reproductive health impacts of exposure to toxic environmental chemicals," *Int J Gynaecol Obstet.* 131, no. 3 (2015): 219-225, DOI: 10.1016/j.ijgo.2015.09.002.

9. Case J—see reference #6.

10. Cambridge Dictionary, Explanation of "incubation." https://dictionary.cambridge.org/us/dictionary/english/incubation. Accessed July 1, 2020.

11. Temkin A, Naidenko O, "Glyphosate Contamination in Food Goes Far Beyond Oat Products. The Environmental Working Group," Feb. 28, 2019. https://www.ewg.org/news-and-analysis/2019/02/glyphosate-contamination-food-goes-far-beyond-oat-products. Accessed July 1, 2020.

12. Samsel A, Seneff S, "Glyphosate pathways to modern diseases VI: Prions, amyloidoses and autoimmune neurological diseases," *Journal of Biological Physics and Chemistry 17 (*2017): 8–32.

13. Frontline. Industrial Meat. *Frontline.* n.d. https://www.pbs.org/wgbh/pages/frontline/shows/meat/industrial/. Accessed July 2, 2020.

14. McKenna, M, *Plucked!: The Truth About Chicken*, London: Little, Brown (February 1, 2018). Available on Amazon: https://www.amazon.com/Plucked-Truth-Chicken-Maryn-McKenna/dp/1408707926/ref=sr_1_3?crid=1G4PB4T6U3LR2&keywords=big+chicken+maryn+mckenna&qid=1575825355&s=books&sprefix=Big+Chicken,stripbooks,124&sr=1-3.

15. Pope, S, "The Real Reason Wheat is Toxic (it's not the gluten)," *The Healthy Home Economist.* n.d. https://www.thehealthyhomeeconomist.com/real-reason-for-toxic-wheat-its-not-gluten/. Accessed July 2, 2020.

16. Milan, O, "Weedkiller found in wide range of breakfast foods aimed at children," *The Guardian*, Aug. 16, 2018. https://www.theguardian.com/environment/2018/aug/16/weedkiller-cereal-monsanto-round-up-childrens-food. Accessed July 2, 2020.

17. Tennant JL, *Healing is Voltage: The Handbook*, 3rd edition, CreateSpace Independent Publishing Platform. Available on Amazon: https://www.amazon.com/Healing-Voltage-Handbook-Jerry-Tennant/dp/1453649166.

Chapter 13

1. Yoshimizu N, MD, PhD, *The Fourth Treatment for Medical Refugees*, Richway International (2009). Available on Amazon.

2. Osilla EV, Marsidi JL, Sharma S., "Physiology, Temperature Regulation," [Updated 2020 Apr 30], in *StatPearls* [Internet], Treasure Island (FL): StatPearls Publishing (2020). Available from: https://www.ncbi.nlm.nih.gov/books/NBK507838/.

3. National Institute of Diabetes and Digestive and Kidney Diseases, "Hypothyroidism (Underactive Thyroid)," Aug 2016, https://www.niddk.nih.gov/health-information/endocrine-diseases/hypothyroidism. Accessed July 2, 2020.

4. Skjodt NM, Atkar R, Easton PA, "Screening for hypothyroidism in sleep apnea," *American journal of respiratory and critical care medicine 160 (*1999): 732-735.

5. Kharrazian D, "Good thyroid health depends on good gut health," *Kharrazian Resource Center*, Sept 6, 2010. https://drknews.com/good-thyroid-health-depends-on-good-gut-health/. Accessed July 2, 2020.

6. Starr, M, MD, *Type 2 Hypothyroidism: The Epidemic,* New Voice Publication (2013). Available on Amazon.

7. Kharrazian D, "Good thyroid health depends on good gut health," Kharrazian Resource Center, Sept 6, 2010. https://drknews.com/good-thyroid-health-depends-on-good-gut-health/. Accessed July 2, 2020.

8. Mercola, Mercola Homepage. https://www.mercola.com/. Accessed July 2, 2020.

9. FluorideAlert.ORG-Fluoride Action Network, Fluoride Action Network Homepage. http://fluoridealert.org/. Accessed July 2, 2020.

10. Kharrzain D, PhD, *Why Do I Still Have Thyroid Symptoms When My Lab Tests Are Normal?* Elephant Press (2010). Available on Amazon

Chapter 14

1. Wilson JL, ND, DC, *PhD, Adrenal Fatigue: The 21st Century Stress Syndrome,* Smart Publications (2001). Available on Amazon.

2. Cadegiani FA, Kater CE, "Adrenal fatigue does not exist: a systematic review [published correction appears in BMC Endocr Disord. 2016 Nov 16;16(1):63]," *BMC Endocr Disord.* 16, no. 1 (2016): 48, published 2016 Aug 24, DOI: 10.1186/s12902-016-0128-4.

Chapter 15

1. Hoevenaar-Blom MP, Spijkerman AM, Kromhout D, Verschuren WM, "Sufficient sleep duration contributes to lower cardiovascular disease risk in addition to four traditional lifestyle factors: the MORGEN study," *Eur J Prev Cardiol.* 21, no. 11 (2014): 1367-1375, DOI: 10.1177/2047487313493057

2. Biswas A, Oh PI, Faulkner GE, et al., "Sedentary time and its association with risk for disease incidence, mortality, and hospitalization in adults: a systematic review and meta-analysis [published correction appears in *Ann Intern Med.* 2015 Sep 1;163(5):400]," *Ann Intern Med.* 162, no. 2 (2015): 123-132, DOI: 10.7326/M14-1651.

3. Stamatakis E, Gale J, Bauman A, Ekelund U, Hamer M, Ding D, "Sitting Time, Physical Activity, and Risk of Mortality in Adults," *Journal of the American College of Cardiology* 73 (2019): 2062-2072.

4. Centers for Disease Control and Prevention (CDC), "Preventing Weight Gain," last reviewed Jan. 28, 2020. https://www.cdc.gov/healthyweight/prevention/index.html. Accessed July 2, 2020.

5. Centers for Disease Control and Prevention (CDC), *National Diabetes Statistics Report*, last reviewed Feb. 14, 2020. https://www.cdc.gov/diabetes/data/statistics/statistics-report.html?CDC_AA_refVal=https://www.cdc.gov/diabetes/data/statistics-report/deaths-cost.html. Accessed July 2, 2020.

6. American Diabetes Association, *Complications*. n.d. https://www.diabetes.org/diabetes/complications. Accessed July 2, 2020.

7. Paz-Graniel I, Babio N, Mendez I, Salas-Salvadó J, "Association between Eating Speed and Classical Cardiovascular Risk Factors: A Cross-Sectional Study," *Nutrients* 11, no. 1 (2019): 83, published 2019. DOI: 10.3390/nu11010083.

8. Saito M, Shimazaki Y, Nonoyama T, Tadokoro Y, "Number of Teeth, Oral Self-care, Eating Speed, and Metabolic Syndrome in an Aged Japanese Population," *J Epidemiol* 29, no. 1 (2019): 26-32, DOI: 10.2188/jea.JE20170210.

Chapter 16

1. Camacho M, Certal V, Abdullatif J, et al., "Myofunctional Therapy to Treat Obstructive Sleep Apnea: A Systematic Review and Meta-analysis," *Sleep* 38, no. 5 (2015): 669-675, published 2015 May 1, DOI: 10.5665/sleep.4652.

Chapter 17

1. Huang YS, Guilleminault C, "Pediatric obstructive sleep apnea and the critical role of oral-facial growth: evidences," *Front Neurol.* 3 (2013): 184, published 2013 Jan 22, DOI: 10.3389/fneur.2012.00184.

2. Chrcanovic BR, Kisch J, Albrektsson T, Wennerberg A, "Bruxism and dental implant failures: a multilevel mixed effects parametric survival analysis approach," *J Oral Rehabil.* 43, no. 11 (2016): 813-823, DOI: 10.1111/joor.12431.

3. Oksenberg A, Arons E, "Sleep bruxism related to obstructive sleep apnea: the effect of continuous positive airway pressure," *Sleep Med.* 3, no. 6 (2002): 513-515, DOI: 10.1016/s1389-9457(02)00130-2.

Chapter 18

1. McKeown P, "Shut your mouth and change your life," *YouTube*, June 22, 2016. https://youtu.be/mBqGS-vEIs0. Accessed July 2, 2020.

2. Al-Delaimy WK, Manson JE, Willett WC, Stampfer MJ, Hu FB, "Snoring as a risk factor for type II diabetes mellitus: a prospective study," *American journal of epidemiology* 155 (2002): 387-393.

3. Palomäki H, "Snoring and the risk of ischemic brain infarction," *Stroke* 22, no. 8 (1991): 1021-1025, DOI: 10.1161/01.str.22.8.1021.

4. Bhattacharjee R, Kheirandish-Gozal L, Spruyt K, et al., "Adenotonsillectomy outcomes in treatment of obstructive sleep apnea in children: a multicenter retrospective study," *Am J Respir Crit Care Med.* 182, no. 5 (2010): 676-683, DOI: 10.1164/rccm.200912-1930OC.

5. Singh GD, Heit T, Preble D, Chandrashekhar R, "Changes in 3D nasal cavity volume after biomimetic oral appliance therapy in adults," *Cranio* 34 (2016): 6.

6. Wilson L. Food sensitivities, intolerance or allergies, June 2019, LD Wilson Consultants, Inc. https://drlwilson.com/Articles/FOODIN-TOL.htm. Accessed July 2, 2020.

7. The Weston A. Price Foundation, "About the Weston A. Price Foundation." https://www.westonaprice.org/. Accessed July 2, 2020.

8. Park S, "How to Treat Your Sinusitis Without Medications [Podcast 83]," *Doctor Steven Park.* n.d. https://doctorstevenpark.com/sinusitis?ck_subscriber_id=371113750. Accessed July 2, 2020.

9. Hein I, "Vaginal Birth and Breastfeeding Linked to Less Allergy," *Medscape*, Nov. 12, 2019. https://www.medscape.com/viewarticle/921147. Accessed July 2, 2020.

Chapter 19

1. World Health Organization (WHO), "Frequently asked questions - What is the WHO definition of health?" n.d. https://www.who.int/about/who-we-are/frequently-asked-questions. Accessed July 5, 2020.

2. HumanN, "How the Body Makes Nitric Oxide," *HumanN*, Nov. 1, 2017. https://www.humann.com/science/body-makes-nitric-oxide/#-section1. Accessed July 6, 2020.

3. Lundberg J.O.N., Weitzberg E, "Nasal nitric oxide in man," *Thorax 54* (1999): 947-952. https://thorax.bmj.com/content/54/10/947.

4. Akerström S, Mousavi-Jazi M, Klingström J, Leijon M, Lundkvist A, Mirazimi A, "Nitric oxide inhibits the replication cycle of severe acute respiratory syndrome coronavirus," *J Virol*. 79, no. 3 (2005): 1966-1969, DOI: 10.1128/JVI.79.3.1966-1969.2005.

5. Lundberg J.O.N., Weitzberg E, "Nasal nitric oxide in man," 1999.

6. HumanN, "How the Body Makes Nitric Oxide," 2017.

7. Thomas DD, "Breathing new life into nitric oxide signaling: A brief overview of the interplay between oxygen and nitric oxide," *Redox Biol*. 5 (2015): 225-233, DOI: 10.1016/j.redox.2015.05.002.

8. Luboshitzky R, Aviv A, Hefetz A, et al., "Decreased pituitary-gonadal secretion in men with obstructive sleep apnea," *J Clin Endocrinol Metab*. 87, no. 7 (2002): 3394-3398, DOI: 10.1210/jcem.87.7.8663.

9. Torregrossa AC, Aranke M, Bryan NS, "Nitric oxide and geriatrics: Implications in diagnostics and treatment of the elderly," *J Geriatr Cardiol*. 8, no. 4 (2011): 230-242, DOI: 10.3724/SP.J.1263.2011.00230.

10. Shin D, Pregenzer G Jr, Gardin JM, "Erectile dysfunction: a disease marker for cardiovascular disease," *Cardiol Rev*. 19, no. 1 (2011): 5-11, DOI: 10.1097/CRD.0b013e3181fb7eb8

11. Cleveland Clinic, "Sudden Cardiac Death (Sudden Cardiac Arrest)," *Cleveland Clinic*, May 14, 2019. https://my.clevelandclinic.org/health/diseases/17522-sudden-cardiac-death-sudden-cardiac-arrest. Accessed July 6, 2020.

12. Montorsi P, Montorsi F, Schulman CC, "Is Erectile Dysfunction the 'Tip of the Iceberg' of a Systemic Vascular Disorder?" *European Urology* 44 (2003): 352-354.

13. Poirier P, "Exercise, Heart Rate Variability, and Longevity: The Cocoon Mystery?" *Circulation* 129 (2014): 2085-2087.

14. Buteyko Clinic, "Unblock the nose," *Buteyko Clinic*. n.d. https://buteykodvd.com/unblock-the-nose/. Accessed July 7, 2020.

Chapter 20

1. Porges S., "The Polyvagal Theory: Neurophysiological Foundations of Emotions, Attachment, Communication, and Self-regulation," Norton Series on Interpersonal Neurobiology, W.W. Norton, 2011.

2. Levine HJ, Rest heart rate and life expectancy, *J Am Coll Cardiol* 30, no. 4 (1997): 1104-1106, DOI: 10.1016/s0735-1097(97)00246-5.

3. Chen X, Barywani SB, Hansson P, et al., "Impact of changes in heart rate with age on all-cause death and cardiovascular events in 50-year-old men from the general population," *Open Heart* 6 (2019): e000856.

4. Habib N, DC, *Activating Your Vagus: Unleash Your Body's Natural Ability to Heal,* Ulysses Press, 2019. Available on Amazon.

Chapter 21

1. Medscape, "Are You Concerned About Shutdown-Related Weight Gain?" *Medscape*, May 19 (2020). https://www.medscape.com/view-article/930774. Accessed July 7, 2020.

2. Price SA, DDS, "Nutrition and Physical Degeneration," The Weston A. Price Foundation, Jan. 1 (2000). https://www.westonaprice.org/physical/. Accessed July 7, 2020.

3. Chapter 22

4. Habib N, DC, *Activating Your Vagus: Unleash Your Body's Natural Ability to Heal,* Ulysses Press (2019). Available on Amazon.

5. Teitelbaum J, MD, *"From Fatigued to Fantastic!"* Penguin Random House, 2020.

6. Bradberry T, Greaves J, "Emotional Intelligence 2.0 TalentSmart," Har/Dol En edition, June 16, 2009. Available on Amazon.

7. Hanh, TN, *Peace Is Every Step: The Path of Mindfulness*, Bantam (March 1992). Available on Amazon.

8. Ibid.

Chapter 23

1. Danenberg A, DDS, *Is Your Gut Killing You?*: An in-depth guide on the connection between the gut, the mouth, chronic disease, and how to stay healthy, www.drdanenberg.com, July 2020, Available on Amazon.

2. Price SA, DDS, "Nutrition and Physical Degeneration," 8th edition (2009), Price-Pottenger Foundation.

3. The Weston A. Prince Foundation: https://www.westonaprice.org.

4. Fallon S, Enig MG, Dearth M, *Nourishing Traditions: The Cookbook that Challenges Politically Correct Nutrition and Diet Dictocrats*, 2nd revised edition, Newtrends Publishing (2001). Available on Amazon: https://www.amazon.com/Nourishing-Traditions-Challenges-Politically-Dictocrats/dp/0967089735.

5. PPNF, "Pottenger's cats: early epigenetics and implications for your health," Nov. 13, 2014. https://price-pottenger.org/uncategorized/pottengers-cats-early-epigenetics-and-implications-for-your-health/. Accessed July 8, 2020.

6. Lin S, *The Dental Diet: The Surprising Link between Your Teeth, Real Food, and Life-Changing Natural Health*, Hay House Inc., Jan. 9, 2018. Available on Amazon: https://www.amazon.com/Dental-Diet-Surprising-between-Life-Changing/dp/1401953174.

7. Stibich M, "The Best Types of Fish to Avoid Mercury," *Very Well Fit*, April 13, 2020. https://www.verywellfit.com/the-best-types-of-fish-for-health-2223830. Accessed July 8, 2020.

8. Myers A. "Collagen and Gelatin: What's the Difference?" *Amy Myers MD*, July 1, 2020. https://www.amymyersmd.com/article/benefits-gelatin-collagen/. Accessed July 8, 2020.

9. Myers A, "9 Signs You Have a Leaky Gut," *Amy Myers MD*, July 1, 2020. https://www.amymyersmd.com/article/signs-leaky-gut/. Accessed July 8, 2020.

10. Cleveland Clinic, "The Best Way You Can Get More Collagen," Cleveland Clinic, May 15, 2018. https://health.clevelandclinic.org/the-best-way-you-can-get-more-collagen/. Accessed July 8, 2020.

11. Brady S, Nurtured Bones homepage. https://nurturedbones.com/. Accessed July 8, 2020.

12. Brady S, Video on bone broth. https://www.facebook.com/nurtured-bones/videos/844794606004879/. Accessed July 8, 2020.

13. Eske J, "What are the benefits of eating Brazil nuts?" *Medical News Today.* n.d. https://www.medicalnewstoday.com/articles/325000. Accessed July 8, 2020.

14. Anarson A, "Walnuts 101: Nutrition Facts and Health Benefits," *Healthline*, Mar. 26, 2019. https://www.healthline.com/nutrition/foods/walnuts. Accessed July 8, 2020.

Chapter 24

1. Liao, F., *Early Sirens,* 2017.

2. Gates D, Food Combining Principles: https://bodyecology.com/food-combiningchart/.

3. Dominguez J, Robin V, *Your Money or Your Life: Transforming Your Relationship with Money and Achieving Financial Independence*, 1999 edition, Penguin Books (1999).

4. Marie-Pierre St-Onge, et al., "*Meal Timing and Frequency: Implications for Cardiovascular Disease Prevention*: A Scientific Statement From the American Heart Association and On behalf of the American Heart Association Obesity Committee of the Council on Lifestyle and Cardiometabolic Health; Council on Cardiovascular Disease in the Young; Council on Clinical Cardiology; and Stroke Council." *Circulation* 135 (2017): e96–e121.

5. Fung, J MD, "The Complete Guide to Fasting: Heal Your Body Through Intermittent, Alternate-Day, and Extended Fasting," 1ˢᵗ edition, Victory Belt Publishing (October 18, 2016). Available on Amazon.

Chapter 25

1. Wahls T, Terry Wahls M.D. Homepage. https://terrywahls.com/start/. Accessed July 8, 2020.

2. Brown R, Kuk JL. Ruth E. Brown, Arya M. Sharma, Chris I. Ardern, Pedi Mirdamadi, Paul Mirdamadi and Jennifer L. Kuk, "Secular differences in the association between caloric intake, macronutrient intake, and physical activity with obesity," *Obesity Research & Clinical Practice* 10 (2015/16): 102.

3. WebMD, "Things That Raise Your Chances of Dementia," WebMD. n.d. https://www.webmd.com/alzheimers/ss/slideshow-raise-chances-dementia. Accessed July 8, 2020.

4. Brauser D, "Sleep Disturbance May Predict Rapid Cognitive Decline in AD," Medscape, May 22, 2020. https://www.medscape.com/viewarticle/931031. Accessed July 8, 2020.

5. Lakhan SE, "Alzheimer Disease," *Medscape*, May 09, 2019. https://emedicine.medscape.com/article/1134817-overview. Accessed July 8, 2020.

Afterword

1. 360 Summits, Holistic Sleep Summit March 5 - March 8 (passed event). https://360summits.com/summit/holistic-sleep-summit/. Accessed July 8, 2020.

Made in United States
Cleveland, OH
24 January 2025